PSYCHEDELIC DRUG TREATMENTS

PSYCHEDELIC DRUG TREATMENTS

Assisting the Therapeutic Process

Dr. Ben Sessa

Eileen Worthley

MERCURY LEARNING AND INFORMATION

Dulles, Virginia | Boston, Massachusetts | New Delhi

Portions of this book were published in *The Psychedelic Renaissance: Reassessing the Role of Psychedelic Drugs in 21st Century Psychiatry and Society.* ISBN: 978-1908995001
Copyright ©2013 by Muswell Hill Press.

Publisher: David Pallai
MERCURY LEARNING AND INFORMATION
22841 Quicksilver Drive
Dulles, VA 20166
info@merclearning.com
www.merclearning.com
(800) 232-0223

This book is printed on acid-free paper.

Dr. Ben Sessa and Eileen Worthley. *Psychedelic Drug Treatments: Assisting the Therapeutic Process.*
ISBN: 9781936420445

Library of Congress Control Number: 2015957710

16 17 18 3 2 1   Printed in the United States of America

Contents

CHAPTER 7 *Promising Research Grinds to a Halt*

PART THREE **Current Research**

CHAPTER 8 *Making Pharmaceuticals Legally Available*

Preface

Picture a cartoon with "thought" bubbles above the heads of several characters. Each of the bubbles encloses a big question mark, and the characters' expressions are askance with disbelief, bewilderment, doubt, skepticism—especially skepticism. These are the looks I encountered when I mentioned the topic or title of this book. "Huh? Psychedelics? You mean, like, LSD? Those are still illegal, aren't they? Wasn't that heyday back in the 1960s? Why would anyone mess around with that stuff nowadays?"

Generally, misinformed or ill-informed folks hold a decidedly negative view of the very concept of using psychedelics to treat any kind of medical or psychiatric condition. Too dangerous, too weird, too outdated hippie-ish, too radical.

Oh? Perhaps electric shock therapy (EST) is less radical? Or lobotomies, maybe they are less dangerous? Modern, legally prescribed antidepressants and antipsychotics—with all their possible side effects—are they any less harmful?

Psychedelic Drug Treatments: Assisting the Therapeutic Process provides information about current and quite viable investigation into reviving and progressing with neurological research that began in the middle of the 20th century and was brought to a halt when the drugs were banned in the 1970s. A remarkable amount of research had been going on before psychedelics became the focus of the War on Drugs and President Richard Nixon declared Timothy Leary to be "the most dangerous man in America." This text will discuss the history of the earlier research efforts and will examine the likelihood of a resurgence of interest in the successful development of methods and practices of clinical therapy assisted by psychedelic drugs.

The purpose of this volume is to promote an understanding of the use of psychedelics as tools to assist therapy and to challenge the 40-year-old prejudices against research into the possible benefits of these drugs.

With technological advances for medical research—such as brain image scanning; fMRI, PET, CT, MRI—available today, neurologists can see what is going on in the live brain. The effects that chemicals have on the brain are no longer subject entirely to conjecture; a scan is a graphic display that is difficult to refute. For example, a scan can show the path that MDMA makes in the brain to disrupt the "fight-or-flight" response that is symptomatic of PTSD. Modern science is ready, willing, and able to observe, record, document, and process information culminating from studies of these drugs on the human brain; it is with the hope of opening minds that are closed to the legality of psychedelics for research that this work is published.

The following pages will introduce you to the way in which the chemical compounds known as psychedelics affect the brain, provide you with the definitions of key terms particular to the neurological and psychological vocabulary, describe the specific disorders that can realistically be helped or relieved through treatment with psychedelics, and offer information with regard to current research being conducted in the field.

I am not a neuroscientist, so I sincerely thank Dr. Ben Sessa, author of *The Psychedelic Renaissance: Reassessing the Role of Psychedelic Drugs in 21st Century Psychiatry and Society*, for contributions from his original work.

Thank you,
Eileen F. Worthley

Acknowledgments

I would like to thank Jennifer Blaney, the project manager at Mercury Learning and Information, for her assistance through the production process of *Psychedelic Drug Treatments: Assisting the Therapeutic Process*. Jen, you so patiently answered my questions and clarified confusion! I appreciate your help and all the work you did on your end.

To David Pallai, founder of Mercury Learning and Information, I am so grateful for the opportunity you gave me to crawl out of my comfort zone, and I thank you for not giving up on me. You have the patience of a saint.

PSYCHEDELIC DRUG TREATMENTS

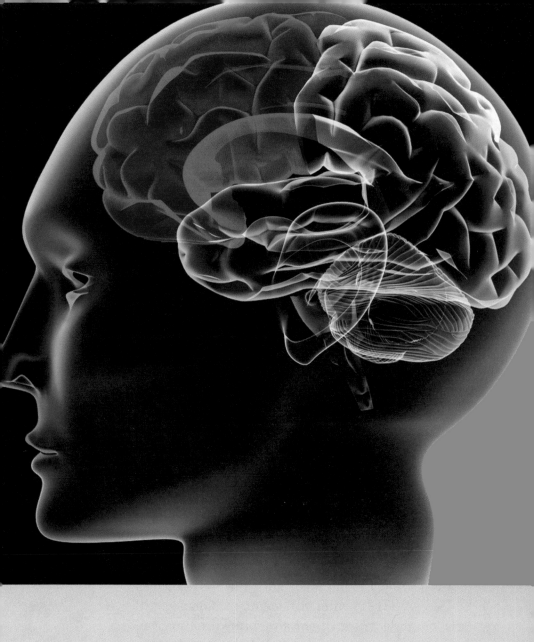

PART ONE

An Introduction to Psychotropic and Psychedelic Drugs

In Chapters 1 and 2 of Part I, we introduce the broad class of compounds known as psychotropic drugs; we will define the terms *psychotropic* and *psychedelic* and will describe the distinctions between the two.

Chapter 3, "A Bit About the Brain," provides definitions of frequently used key terms particular to the neurological and psychological vocabulary.

Chapter 4, "How Do Psychoactive Medications Work in the Brain?" will offer an easily comprehensible explanation of the way these chemical compounds act in the brain.

CHAPTER 1
Psychoactive Compounds

CHAPTER 2
Psychedelic Compounds

CHAPTER 3
A Bit About the Brain

CHAPTER 4
How Do Psychoactive Medications Work in the Brain?

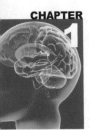

Psychoactive Compounds

Psychedelics are considered to be part of a wider class of chemical compounds known as psychoactive drugs. Although the primary purpose of this text is to offer information about psychedelic drug therapy specifically, it will be helpful to first discuss the class of psychoactive drugs generally, because many of these medicines are legally and commonly prescribed to treat psychiatric disorders. The intention of the authors throughout this text is to provide information to promote the opinion that several psychiatric conditions could potentially benefit to a greater degree from treatment with psychedelic compounds, which are, as of this writing, neither legal nor common.

As you embark on your trip through the pages of this text, we urge you to watch Part 1 of a film titled *Psychedelic Drugs– The Unexplained.* This video will serve as an introduction to the world of psychedelic research for use in psychiatric therapy and the goal of this text, which is to encourage a legal renewal of those efforts.

ON THE WEB

http://www.youtube.com/watch? v=XtB8SUlaM8g

1. What are psychoactive drugs?

Beware! There are a lot of "psychos" out there—lurking on the shelves at your local pharmacy—stuffed in pockets, hanging around on street corners—hiding in night tables and in medicine chests—and synthesizing in laboratories around the world. It's important to know what the terms mean, and because they are frequently used somewhat interchangeably, we will draw some distinctions.

- Psychoactive: affecting the mind or behavior (1959)
- Psychotropic: acting on the mind (1948)
- Psychotherapeutic: relating to or involving psychotherapy (1854)
- Psychoanalytic: of or relating to psychoanalysis (1906)
- Psychopharmaceutical: a drug having an effect on the mental state of the user (1962)

Psychoactive compounds are a broad spectrum of chemical substances that impact the central nervous system, affecting the areas in the brain that control mood and behavior; sometimes these drugs alter perception and consciousness. Many psychoactive chemicals are naturally occurring substances (organic

4   PART ONE | *An Introduction to Psychotropic and Psychedelic Drugs*

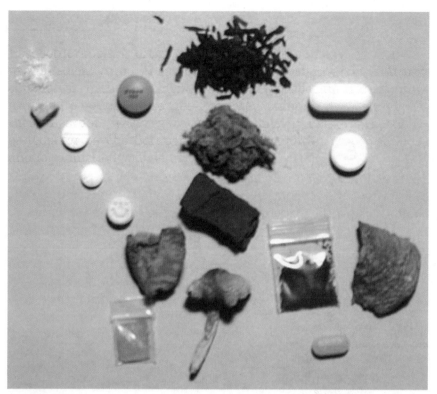

▲ FIGURE 1.1

An arrangement of psychoactive drugs including (counter-clockwise from top left): cocaine, crack, methylphenidate (Ritalin), ephedrine, MDMA (Ecstasy: lavender pill with smile), mescaline (green dried cactus flesh), LSD (2 × 2 blotter in tiny baggie), psilocybin (dried Psilocybe cubensis mushroom), Salvia divinorum (10X extract in small baggie), diphenhydramine (Benadryl: pink pill), Amanita muscaria (red dried mushroom cap piece), Tylenol #3 (contains codeine), codeine containing muscle relaxant, pipe tobacco (top), bupropion (Zyban: brownish-purple pill), cannabis (green bud center), hashish (brown rectangle).

compounds) found in plants and herbs, fungi and molds, and in the central nervous systems of some animals. They range from relatively benign (the chocolate-producing cacao bean or caffeine-producing coffee bean) to profoundly perception altering (the fungus *ergot*, which produces lysergic acid—a main component of LSD). Further, many of these substances mimic the naturally occurring chemicals in our own systems. Figure 1.1 shows an assortment of psychoactive drugs, including mass-produced psychopharmaceuticals and natural substances. How these chemicals work is covered in a little more depth in "A Bit About the Brain."

2. How are psychotropic drugs different from psychoactive drugs?

The terms psychoactive and **psychotropic** are frequently used interchangeably, which is understandable, given that their meanings are so similar; the fine line of distinction between them is that psychotropic drugs are *prescribed* for the purpose of interacting with the natural chemicals in the brain; they can elevate or stabilize mood, control erratic behavior, alleviate anxiety. Psychotropic drugs, then, are a subset of psychoactive compounds; all psychotropics are psychoactive, but not all psychoactives are psychotropic. For example, in our introductory paragraph, caffeine is mentioned as a relatively mild psychoactive; cocaine is a much stronger and potentially more dangerous drug. Though coffee might make one feel bright-eyed and perky, and cocaine can make one feel an on-top-of-the-world confidence, neither of these would be prescribed to affect mood, cognition, or behavior; so they are examples of psychoactive but *not* psychotropic substances. Antidepressants, however, are prescribed to deliberately effect changes in mood by working in harmony with a body's natural chemical makeup. Antidepressants, mood stabilizers, antianxiety medications, ADHD drugs, and antipsychotics are among the more common types of psychotropic drugs prescribed by doctors, as well as pain relievers and anesthetics. Many of these legally dispensed medications are further classified as **psychotherapeutic**.

A series of very brief and easy-to-follow video lessons on "Consciousness" at udacity.com offers descriptions, explanations, and definitions. Starting with "What is a drug?" at https://www.udacity.com/course/viewer#!/c-ps001/l-233544439/e-233198861/m-233198862, the lessons progress one after another, some ending with a simple question or quiz that reinforces understanding. A lesson or quiz can be skipped or repeated by hovering the cursor over the sections of the bar at the top of the page where topics are displayed "Psychoactive and Psychotropic" is explained rather well at https://www.udacity.com/course/viewer#!/c-ps001/l-233544439/m-233198872.

An overview of lesson topics is presented at "Exploring aspects of drugs" at https://www.udacity.com/course/viewer#!/c-ps001/l-233544439/m-233198866.

Psychotherapeutic drugs are psychotropic substances that are used medically and in conjunction with psychotherapy and psychoanalysis in the treatment of symptoms of specific mental, physical, and emotional disorders. In later chapters, we will discuss these disorders with regard to the viability of using psychedelics as tools for psychotherapeutic use—to enhance therapy sessions and for addiction counseling.

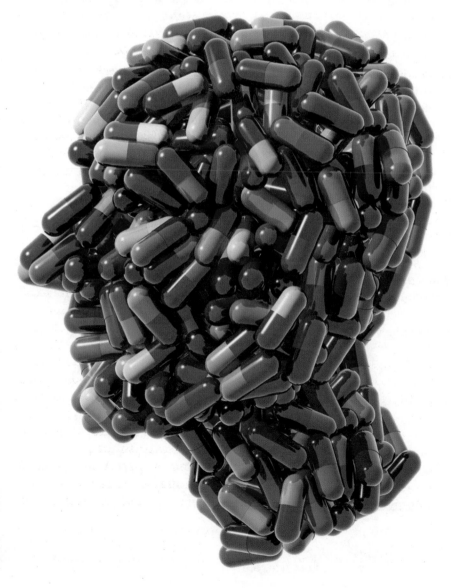

4. How are psychopharmaceuticals distinguished from the other "psychos"?

Just as "psychotropic drugs" are a subset of psychoactive drugs, **psychopharmaceuticals** can be considered a subset of psychotropics. These medications are synthetic drugs, developed by researchers and pharmaceutical companies, which are used to effect changes in mood and behavior.

Because this text will deal specifically with psychedelic compounds, we will not provide detailed information about these types of psychotherapeutic medications and the disorders they are used to treat; however, brief general descriptions follow as an introduction to further discussion of the similarities and differences between these regularly prescribed drugs and the class of psychoactives known as psychedelics.

5. What are some psychotherapeutic medications and what disorders do they treat?

- **Antidepressants** interact with the natural chemicals in the brain called **neurotransmitters**, which affect mood, emotions, feelings of anxiety, and general frame of mind. Major depression is a chronic illness that is characterized by a persistent, unshakable feeling of sadness, low sense of self-esteem, and loss of interest in pleasurable activities; although depression is a psychiatric illness, it frequently causes physical symptoms.

> "Major depressive disorder affects approximately 14.8 million American adults, or about 6.7 percent of the US population age 18 and older in a given year."
>
> *http://www.nimh.nih.gov/health/ publications/the-numbers-count-mental-disorders-in-america/index.shtml*

Mood stabilizers are also used to treat **major depressive disorder** and **dysthymic disorder** (chronic, mild, prolonged depression), but they are more specifically used to treat **bipolar disorder**, also known as manic-depressive disorder. Although major depression is one trait of bipolar disorder, it is further characterized by extreme swings in mood that shift from depression to manic behavior.

- **Antianxiety medications** are used—sometimes in conjunction with antidepressants—to treat the following anxiety and stress-related disorders:

- Obsessive-compulsive disorder (OCD)
- Posttraumatic stress disorder (PTSD)
- Generalized anxiety disorder (GAD)
- Panic disorder
- Social anxiety disorder
- Specific phobias

- **ADHD drugs** are predominantly stimulants used to treat **Attention Deficit Hyperactivity Disorder**. Although more common in children, ADHD also affects many adults. These specific stimulants are presumed to increase the level of dopamine, which is a neurotransmitter responsible for regulating attention and movement.

- **Antipsychotic medications** are used to treat schizophrenia and related mental health disorders that include hallucinations, delusions, and psychoses. These psychopharmaceuticals decrease the amount of anxiety and agitation that is a typical trait of schizophrenia; they also decrease cognitive impairment (difficulty in concentrating and remembering) and they can control delusions and psychotic episodes. Some of these medications have been available since the middle of the 20th century, with varying degrees of success; they are known as **first-generation antipsychotics** and include what are considered to be the conventional, "typical" antipsychotics. The typical antipsychotics interact with the dopamine neurotransmitters that control

DEFINITION Bipolar disorder, also known as manic-depressive illness, is a brain disorder that causes unusual shifts in mood, energy, activity levels, and the ability to carry out day-to-day tasks. Symptoms of bipolar disorder are severe. They are different from the normal ups and downs that everyone goes through from time to time. Bipolar disorder symptoms can result in damaged relationships, poor job or school performance, and even suicide.

http://www.nimh.nih.gov/health/topics/bipolar-disorder/index.shtml

NOTE According to the National Institute of Mental Health (NIMH), psychiatric medications treat mental disorders. Sometimes called psychotropic or psychotherapeutic medications, they have changed the lives of people with mental disorders for the better. Many people with mental disorders live fulfilling lives with the help of these medications. Without them, people with mental disorders might suffer serious and disabling symptoms . . . Medications treat the symptoms of mental disorders. They cannot cure the disorder, but they make people feel better so they can function.

movement, so a common side effect is interference with motor control, which can be as moderate as a slight feeling of restlessness or tremors to as severe as a condition called tardive kinesia, which causes unusual and uncontrollable body movements or tics. **Second-generation antipsychotics** (SGAs) came into development in the 1990s and are considered as "atypical" because they act on the serotonin receptors as well as the dopamine pathways, so they do not cause the same side effects as the first-generation medications, particularly with regard to body movement challenges. SGAs can, however, cause weight gain and diabetes in some people.

Several of these illnesses and conditions will be discussed again in later chapters on research into the use of psychedelic drugs in the therapeutic treatment of specific psychiatric disorders.

To learn more about these classes of psychotropic drugs and the psychiatric disorders they treat, there is a wealth of information, including names of specific medications, descriptions of possible side effects, psychiatric uses and benefits, and cautionary advisories issued by the Food and Drug Administration as published by the National Institute for Mental Health:

http://www.nimh.nih.gov/health/ publications/mental-health-medications/ index.shtml

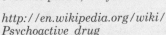
6. How long have these medicines been used therapeutically?

"There is archaeological evidence of the use of psychoactive substances (mostly plants) dating back at least 10,000 years, and historical evidence of cultural use over the past 5,000 years."

http://en.wikipedia.org/wiki/ Psychoactive_drug

As mentioned, many psychoactive compounds are unsynthesized and occur naturally in plants, mushrooms, cacti, and molds.

It is widely accepted that humankind has been ingesting these compounds for several thousands of years, dating back to prehistoric times.

Early "patent" medications claiming to be rendered from exotic ingredients have been sold since as early as the 17th century, and the early days of the advertising industry promoted medicines as one of the first major products.

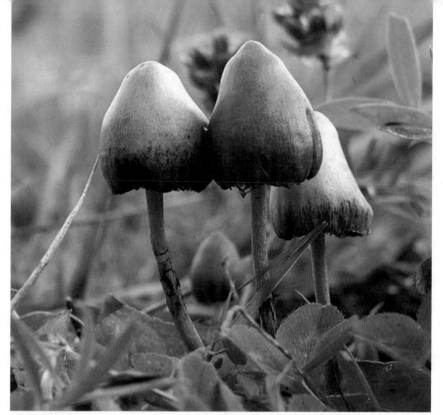

▲ **FIGURE 1.2**
Psychoactive compounds occur naturally in several psilocybin mushroom species.
This mushroom is called "Liberty Cap" (Psilocybe semilanceata).
SOURCE: © 2007 Arp, image number 6514 at Mushroom Observer. *http://upload.wikimedia
.org/wikipedia/commons/4/4a/Psilocybe_semilanceata_6514.jpg*

▶ **FIGURE 1.3**
Typical patent medicine label.

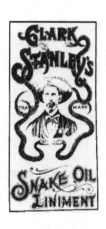

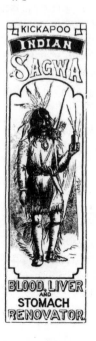

Little seems to have changed in that today's pharmaceutical companies assume a significant share of advertising space and time.

7. What are designer drugs?

There are a significant and growing number of readily available psychopharmaceuticals known as research chemicals (RCs) or **designer drugs**. These psychoactive compounds are offshoots of existing drugs, formulated through minor modifications to the structure and composition of well-known psychoactive substances. In the late 1990s and early 2000s, the Internet provided an ideal marketplace for the manufacturers of designer drugs to sell their products. The term and concept of "research chemicals" was coined by some vendors (in particular, sellers of psychedelic drugs) who believed that selling the chemicals for "scientific research" rather than human consumption would sidestep a section of the **US Controlled Substances Act** (CSA; 1970) called the **Federal Analogue Act** (also called the Alcohol and Drug Abuse Amendments of 1986 or the Anti-Drug Abuse Act of 1986). The term "analogue" in this sense refers to a chemical compound that is structurally similar to another but differs slightly in composition. Vendors of designer drugs attempted to take advantage of a clause in the Act that specified that any chemical "substantially similar" to a Schedule I or II controlled substance should be considered as if it were also listed in those schedules, *but only if intended for human consumption.* In 2004, several of these Internet-based vendors and two manufacturers were shut down in a **US Drug Enforcement Administration (DEA)** operation called "Web Tryp."

Many designer drugs are still available through the black market, but most are too recently developed to have undergone sufficient study to determine their modes of action or their effects on the human body. This text, therefore, will discuss the more commonly known psychotropic drugs, about which a considerable amount of data has been gathered over several decades of research; the intent of this book is to convey information that will promote the development of psychedelics into accepted, viable psychotherapeutic medicines.

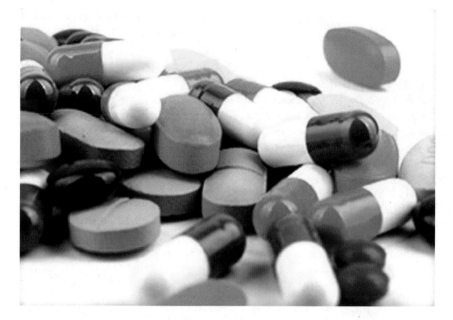

In this chapter, we offered some general information about various types of drugs—and we met some "psychos"! Our next chapter will deal more specifically with the psychedelics.

Psychedelic Compounds

CHAPTER 2

8. What are psychedelic drugs?

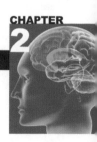

DEFINITION

A **psychedelic drug** is a psychoactive substance that, when ingested, alters perception and consciousness.

As mentioned previously, psychedelics are one of several classes of psychoactives. Together with **dissociatives** and **deliriants**, psychedelics make up the class of psychoactive compounds known as **hallucinogens**, which induce varying states of altered consciousness. The perceptual illusions induced by the use of psychedelics can be profound and can affect all of the sensory modalities. The nature of these illusions is somewhat different from the **hallucinations** experienced by using dissociatives and deliriants, however, and it is important to realize the differences among the drug types. The use of psychedelics is associated

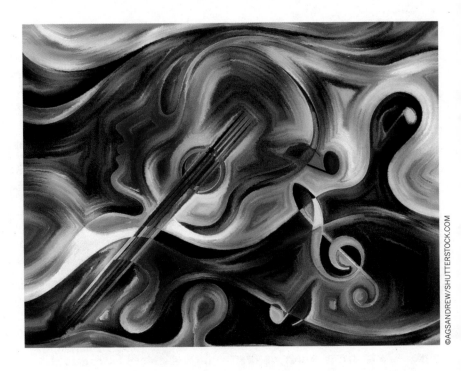

with a desire to expand one's mind to embrace experiences of an unusually spiritual and uplifting nature, to enhance creative thought, to come to a better understanding of "self" in relationship with the universe. The psychedelics create distortions of something that exists in the reality of the present and immediate physical or conscious environment of the person who has taken the drug. For example, if one is listening to music, one might imagine "seeing" the music as colors swirling around, and one might feel so completely enveloped by the colors and the sounds that he or she perceives him- or herself to be not a mere audience to the music but to be *in* the music *as a part* of the sounds and the colors.

9. How are psychedelics different from other hallucinogens?

It is a bit misleading and something of a misnomer to classify psychedelics as **hallucinogens** (please see definitions), because there is *no complete break from reality*. Psychedelics create **illusions**, altered perceptions of the true environment; many other hallucinogens create **delusions** and entirely false perceptions. A user knows that he or she is under the influence of a psychedelic and that the effects will wear off. He or she will possibly see ordinary objects—animal, vegetable, and mineral—in extraordinary, colorful, shape-changing ways, but the user is still aware of the reality of the environment.

Dissociatives, as the name implies, make one feel *disassociated* from his or her surroundings. The detached self becomes depersonalized, and the usual harmony of consciousness, memory, personal identity, and perception of surroundings and other people becomes disrupted. Dissociatives can be effectively used as anesthetics because the "self" is "gone" and is insensible to pain. At high doses, dissociatives can induce catalepsy and even amnesia.

Deliriants induce a state of *delusion* and *delirium*, extreme confusion, and an inability to control one's actions. These drugs can cause a complete disconnect from reality that is comparable to that experienced by people who suffer from schizophrenia and severe psychoses.

Hallucination: a completely unfounded or mistaken impression or notion; a delusion

Illusion: perception of something objectively existing in such a way as to cause or permit misinterpretation of its actual nature either because of the ambiguous qualities of the thing perceived or because of the personal characteristics of the one perceiving or because of both factors

Delusion: a false belief regarding the self or persons or objects outside the self that persists despite the facts and is common in paranoia, schizophrenia, and psychotic depressed states

The kinds of illusions experienced through psychedelics are well described in many of the songs of the psychedelic era. A few phrases from *Lucy in the Sky with Diamonds* by John Lennon and Paul McCartney (1967) are quoted here; the entire song (and a video) can be heard at *http://www.youtube.com/watch?v=ZqXmBy1_qOQ*

On psychedelics, the mind expands to imbue objects, people, and environment with unseen-before qualities.

> Picture yourself in a boat on a river with tangerine trees and marmalade skies,
> Somebody calls you, you answer quite slowly, a girl with kaleidoscope eyes.
> Cellophane flowers of yellow and green, towering over your head . . .
> Follow her down to a bridge by a fountain, where rocking horse people
> eat marshmallow pies.
> Everyone smiles as you drift past the flowers that grow so incredibly high . . .
>
> —Lennon & McCartney, 1967

Trees and sky could be perceived to change colors (tangerine and marmalade), but one would not suffer the delusion of a tree suddenly springing up where there is none. Looking into the face of a friend, one might see his or her eyes as multicolored, changing

For a live subject's reaction to taking LSD, there is rare footage (8–9 min.) of a film made in the 1950s. The user is a housewife, and she volunteered to participate in the LSD experiment.

https://www.youtube.com/watch?v=BTjRi0 x2Cyg&list=PL709ufoAtf4fvTCm2m6bSRpt H2JUHMAHE&index=9

A well-informed, recently made, 55-minute documentary (from National Geographic Explorer) on LSD can be watched at *https://www.youtube.com/ watch?v=14WtwJTwuWg.*

This film covers some history and discusses present efforts to perform research with LSD. It includes comments from people who have participated in studies and experiments with psychedelics.

patterns; but one doesn't visualize a person who is not really there. On psychedelics, there is an energy—a life force—that surrounds and joins the user with natural phenomena that are present. To borrow words from another Lennon–McCartney (1967) song—"life flows on within you and without you." One feels so intensely connected to natural surroundings that he or she feels a part of them. Flowers might be intensely colorful and they might be imagined to grow "incredibly high" because one feels in tune with them in a cellular way. One might feel a sense of time slowing, or even stopping, and a feeling of drifting along with the energy that evokes a sense of "oneness."

10. What does "psychedelic" mean?

Doctor Humphry Osmond, a British psychiatrist and researcher practicing in Canada, publicly introduced the term "psychedelic" at a meeting of the New York Academy of Sciences in 1957, and it is the term that has been adopted by both the research community and popular culture.

Phantastica. First published in 1924, *Phantastica: Narcotic and Stimulating Drugs* is the title of a book by German pharmacologist Louis Lewin, who was one of the first scientists to recognize that the pharmacology of various plants created different and specific mental effects when ingested.

The word "psychedelic," which was first used in 1957, literally means "mind manifesting." Psychedelics tend to affect the mind in a way that allows the conscious to explore one's surroundings or thoughts with heightened awareness and sensitivity; the mind is able to manifest a deep or enlightened manner of contemplation that is unusually dissimilar to the ordinary conscious state.

Before the term "psychedelic" was popularly accepted, **phantastica, psychotomimetic, phanerothyme,** and **psycholytic** were terms used to identify these particular, peculiar compounds.

11. What do these alternative terms mean?

Lewin classified various psychoactive drugs based on their psychoactive effects, bringing new words into popular usage. His categories included the **euphoriants**, such as heroin; the **inebriants**, such as alcohol; and the class of drugs he named **phantastica**, which later became known as the psychedelics.

12. What are the various psychedelic compounds?

Most psychedelic drugs are categorized as one of two types of chemical compounds: **tryptamines** or **phenethylamines**, which are both naturally occurring chemical compounds. Tryptamine is found in plants, fungi, and animals (particularly the jaguar); much is not yet known about tryptamines, but it is believed that they act as neurotransmitters, found in trace amounts in the brains of mammals. Most psychedelic drugs with acronyms ending in T are tryptamines. Phenethylamine (also spelled phenylethylamine) is found in plant and animal enzymes and functions as a neuromodulator in the central nervous system of mammals. It is also found in many other organisms and foods, such as chocolate; its chemical structure is similar to that of many naturally occurring amphetamines and stimulants. Close relatives of both tryptamine and phenethylamine are found in their natural states in high concentrations in our brains, and it is speculated by some

NOTE Lewin's study marked a turning point in the field of ethnobotany (the study of relationships between people and plants). Books had been written about how people used these mind-altering plants, but Lewin's was the first to examine how the plants produced their various effects. "*Phantastica* was the first book to bring scientific insights to a survey of the use of drugs around the world."

http://www.amazon.com/Phantastica-Classic-Survey-Mind-Altering-Plants/dp/0892817836

DEFINITION **Psychotomimetic.** In the late 1940s, it was thought that psychedelics were valuable tools for the study of psychoses. Researchers and clinicians at that time believed that these drugs could mimic psychotic episodes and that, by ingesting the drugs themselves, they would more keenly understand what it is like to be schizophrenic; this type of study fostered the term "psychotomimetic," in other words, "to mimic psychoses."

DEFINITION **Phanerothyme.** It was writer Aldous Huxley who, in the early 1950s, coined the term "phanerothyme," which means "to make the soul visible," after taking mescaline and feeling an undeniable spiritual enlightenment as a significant part of his experience:

"To make this trivial world sublime
Take half a gramme of phanerothyme."

researchers that it is possible that endogenous psychedelic chemicals are secreted by our brains under ordinary, apparently nonpsychedelic, circumstances. For example, the common and immensely important neurotransmitter serotonin 5-hydroxytryptamine (5-HT) is the base molecule tryptamine with an extra oxygen molecule. Dimethlytryptamine (DMT) is an extremely potent psychedelic substance that is simply the same tryptamine structure but with two extra carbon atoms instead of the oxygen molecule. Both are extremely close to tryptamine structurally, but they have dramatically different effects on the brain.

13. What are the effects of the tryptamine-based psychedelics?

Tryptamine-based psychedelics are thought to be the more disorienting in terms of consciousness-altering illusions. Generally— and it is important to understand and remember that effects vary from person to person, dosage to dosage, and setting to setting—tryptamine-based psychedelics can distort visual and auditory sensory perceptions and can produce intense feelings of euphoria, love, spirituality, and "connectedness" with one's surroundings; muscle relaxation, body heaviness, and dilated pupils are all common physical reactions, and occasionally nausea is experienced.

Descriptions in the following lists are, for the most part, obtained from the Erowid (which loosely means "Earth Wisdom") website at *www.erowid.org/chemicals/*. Erowid.org is a noncommercial, nonprofit, online library dedicated to providing "accurate, specific, and responsible information" about psychoactive plants, drugs, and chemicals. The Vaults of Erowid are well established (since 1994), containing more than 50,000 documents, images, research summaries and abstracts, media reports, and experiential anecdotes to educate the site visitor on the pharmacology, history, effects, chemistry, legality, politics, and cultural aspects of hundreds of psychoactive substances. Information contributors include doctors, researchers, chemists, teachers, lawyers, therapists, and health professionals.

ON THE WEB

14. What are the tryptamine psychedelics?

Following is a list of the more well-known tryptamine-based psychedelic drugs, with very brief descriptions. The more widely researched compounds from this list will be treated in more detail in later chapters as we explore their psychotherapeutic benefits.

- **LSD** is the most well-known and most researched psychedelic. Although in its synthesized form it is relatively new compared to magic mushrooms and peyote buttons, which have been available for thousands of years, it is the standard against which all other psychedelics are compared and, considering the relatively miniscule effective dosage, is one of the most potent mood-changing chemicals. It is synthesized from lysergic acid, which is found in the ergot fungus that grows on rye and other grains.
- **Psilocybin** is naturally occurring and obtained from over 200 species of mushrooms collectively known as psilocybin mushrooms, better known as **Magic Mushrooms**. Psilocybin is almost certainly among the first of psychoactive substances known to mankind; the mushrooms were plentiful in the wild and could be (and still can be) eaten "as is"; synthesizing in a chem lab is not required in order to extract the desired drug.
- **Dimethyltryptamine (DMT)**, is a powerful visual psychedelic that produces short-acting effects when smoked. Produced by the pineal gland in the brain, DMT is released during the REM phase of sleep and is thought to produce or affect our dreams.
- **5-MeO-DMT** is a naturally occurring psychedelic present in numerous plants and in the venom of the *Bufo alvarius* toad. It is found in some traditional South American shamanic concoctions and sometimes in ayahuasca brews. It is somewhat comparable in its effects to DMT; however, it is substantially more potent, so it should not be confused with DMT.
- **Bufotenin** is a naturally occurring psychedelic present in many species of plants and in Bufo toad venom. There has been some controversy over the psychoactivity of bufotenin; recent data suggests that it is similar in effects to, though less potent than, 5-MeO-DMT.
- **Ibogaine** is the active chemical found in the African Tabernanthe iboga root as well as several other plant species. It is a strong, long-lasting psychedelic used traditionally in a coming-of-age ritual but also known for its modern use in treating opiate addiction. Ibogaine is

unlike the other compounds listed here in that it can cause very strong hallucinations and can have dissociative effects.

15. What are the effects of the phenethylamine-based psychedelics?

The phenethylamine naturally produced in the central nervous system (beta-phenethylamine) is considered to be the body's own form of amphetamine; phenethylamine-based psychedelics are often considered to be more stimulating, evoking an "adrenaline-rush" sensation. They are considered to be *empathogenic* (inducing empathy) or *entactogenic* (touched from within) substances and commonly intensify feelings of sensuality, empathy, trust, and deeper emotional closeness to people.

16. What are the phenethylamine psychedelics?

The following list of phenethylamine psychedelics includes only those that have been or are the most popular. The 2C compounds at the end of the list are newly created synthetic psychoactives. Although these do not have a lengthy history of use and do not have "street cred," some of these chemicals are being researched for their potential benefit to the field of psychotherapy.

- **MDMA** (3,4-methylenedioxymethamphetamine), more well-known as ecstasy, is one of the most popular recreational psychoactives. It is known for its empathogenic, euphoric, and stimulant effects; it also has been used in psychotherapy.
- **Mescaline** is a naturally occurring psychedelic with a long history of human use. It is the primary active chemical in the peyote cactus; as with the psilocybin mushroom, it has been readily available without needing to be synthesized, it most surely was enjoyed by early man eons before beakers and pipettes were ever thought of.
- **MDA** is a synthetic empathogen sometimes found in ecstasy tablets. It is closely related to MDMA, although its effects are said to be slightly more psychedelic.
- **Mephedrone** is a powerful stimulant and is part of a group of drugs that are closely related to amphetamines, such as speed and ecstasy.

- **2C-B** is a synthetic psychedelic that first gained popularity as a legal Ecstasy replacement in the mid-1980s. It is known for having a strong physical component to its effects and a moderate duration.
- **2C-I** is a short-acting synthetic psychedelic. It gained some popularity in Europe and the United States between 2001 and 2005.
- **2C-T-4** is a synthetic psychedelic. It is very uncommon and has only a short history of human use.
- **2C-T-7** is a synthetic psychedelic known for its colorful visuals. It experienced a surge in popularity, due to Internet sales, during 1999–2001, before becoming illegal in the United States.

The detailed chemistry of these psychedelic drugs and other psychoactive compounds is not the concern of this text; however, those who wish a more in-depth education on the pharmacology of psychedelics are directed to the Erowid site mentioned previously and to two texts by Alexander and Anne Shulgin: *PiHKAL (Phenethylamines i Have Known and Loved)* and *TiHKAL (Tryptamines i Have Known and Loved)*.

These "bibles" of psychoactive substances describe in great detail the psychoactive effects and the chemical construction of hundreds of substances from the very common to those so rare they are merely conceptual. These books include beautifully written stories about the last 50 years of psychedelic history. Chemist Alexander Shulgin has been dubbed "the godfather of MDMA" and remains a much-loved figure in the psychedelic world.

ON THE WEB

An informative video featuring the Shulgins is available at *http://www.youtube.com/watch?v=9kDl-V5RuQo*

In this video, the Shulgins present an understandable explanation of these organic compounds as being basically chemical nuclei upon which any number of substances and medicines can be created by addition, subtraction, and rearrangement of atoms. They also offer their opinions with regard to possible dangerous side effects and the illegal classification of psychedelic drugs.

These first two chapters have explained, basically, what psychoactive and psychedelic substances are. Our next chapter offers definitions of specific terms that will appear throughout this text as we discuss in greater detail the action of psychoactive chemicals in the brain and the research efforts and clinical trials of the psychedelics.

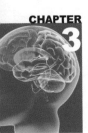

CHAPTER 3

A Bit About the Brain

This chapter and Chapter 4 will offer information about how psychotherapeutic drugs work in the brain. It is not the goal of this text to plunge into the intricacies of neuroscience, but it will be helpful, in order to understand how psychoactives and psychedelics affect the brain, to first have a bit of a basic understanding about the brain itself and to become familiar with a few pertinent neurological and chemical terms that will be used throughout the following pages.

17. How does the brain work?

That's a short and simplistic question for such a vast, complicated subject. Neuroscientists are still exploring the mysteries of an incredibly complicated organ that is responsible for absolutely everything we do, think, and feel. There are some facts that are known, however:

- The human brain is about the size of two fists held together and weighs approximately 3 pounds, accounting for only 2% of the body's total weight.
- Bundled together in the brain are over *100 billion* microscopic cells called **neurons**. (See Figure 3.1.)
- Neurons connect with each other to form an extremely intricate messaging system throughout the head and body; everything about us is controlled by these neurons, and millions of messages are constantly being sent and received by connecting neurons—all of our thoughts, senses, movements, and emotions.
- Each neuron is capable of connecting to—on average—10,000 other neurons; this adds up to over *100 trillion* connections—our brains are very efficient multitaskers!
- There are two major neural networks acting simultaneously; the **central nervous system** and the **peripheral nervous system**. Within these major systems are many subsystems. The central nervous system includes the brain and the spinal column; psychoactive compounds affect the central nervous system. The peripheral nervous system comprises the nerves outside of the brain and spinal column. We will be primarily concerned with the central nervous system, but the

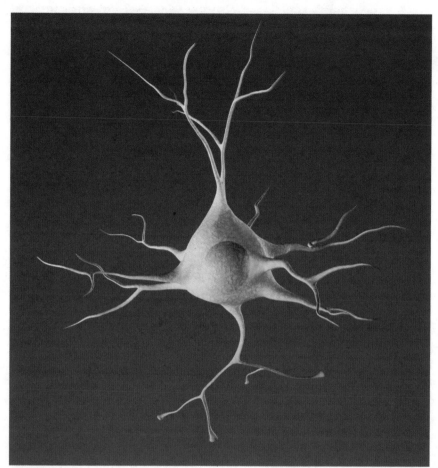

▲ FIGURE 3.1
A single neuron.
SOURCE: Image courtesy of the National Institute on Aging/National Institutes of Health.

importance of the peripheral nervous system is that it acts as a conduit to parts of the body outside of the brain.

- The somatic, or "voluntary," nervous system is able to consider a problem, smell what's cooking, listen to music, feel a sore tooth, type on a keyboard, squint at a screen, answer the

 NOTE The main function of the PNS [peripheral nervous system] is to connect the central nervous system to the limbs and organs, essentially serving as a communication relay going back and forth between the brain and the extremities . . . The peripheral nervous system is divided into the **somatic** nervous system and the **autonomic** nervous system . . . *http://en.wikipedia.org/wiki/ Peripheral_nervous_system*

phone, anticipate what will be going on later in the day, and a multitude of other sensations—all at one time.

- The neural connections of the autonomic nervous system are considered "involuntary"; they function without our conscious thought to control our heartbeat, our breathing, our digestion, our hair growing, our cells renewing, and other bodily functions that we take for granted and barely notice.

There are myriad fascinating details about the neurological wonder that is the human brain, and current technology is helping neuroscientists uncover more details every day. According to *The Human Brain* (see the On the Web icon), more has been discovered about the brain in the last five years than in the last 5,000 years. The focus of our text, however, is on the **neural connections** and the effect of psychoactive drugs and medications on these neural connections.

18. How do the neurons connect to each other?

Neurons are of varying types, shapes, and sizes, depending on what they do, and the manner in which they connect with each other to transmit messages is one aspect of neurological study. The most basic kind of neural connection is through what one might think of as a "door" called a **synapse**.

To explore the brain in more detail, there are two highly recommended, full-length documentaries:

ON THE WEB

The Human Brain is available at *http://www.youtube.com/watch?v=1imN6oc_YtU*
How Does the Brain Work / Nova 1080p HD is available at *http://www.youtube.com/watch?v=lhIJbIX1_D0*
For a shorter video you might enjoy *The Universe Inside Your Head* at *http://www.brainfacts.org/brain-basics/neural-network-function/articles/2013/the-universe-inside-your-head/*
For more detailed but easy-to-follow information and a slideshow of the way the nervous systems interact, see *http://www.mayoclinic.org/brain/SLS-20077047?sl=?&slide=6*

19. What are neurotransmitters?

The chemicals that cross the synaptic cleft are called **neurotransmitters**; you will see this term frequently in the following pages, because it is these chemicals that can be altered—diminished or enhanced—through the use of psychoactive compounds. A neurotransmitter is an endogenous chemical that transmits electrical signals between neurons and other cells in the body.

Figure 3.2 shows the most basic kind of transmission, which is at the synapse (synapses are located at various places along the **dendrite** branches), where neurotransmitters are released from the "message dispatch center," which is called the **axon terminal**, or the **presynaptic** side of the synapse.

The neurotransmitter chemicals are enclosed in packages called **vesicles** under the membrane of the axon terminal and are released to cross the synaptic gap, or cleft, to bind to **receptors** (a receptor is a protein molecule on or inside the cell that receives the chemical signals of the neurotransmitters; the receiving neuron or cell is on the **postsynaptic** side of the synapse), on the other cell or neuron and is conducted through the dendrites to the cell body of the receiving neuron.

A **synapse** is a specialized junction at which a neural cell (neuron) communicates with a target cell. At a synapse, a neuron releases a chemical transmitter that diffuses across a small gap and activates special sites, called **receptors**, on the target cell. The target cell may be another neuron or a specialized region of a muscle or secretory cell. *http://www.medterms.com/script/main/art.asp?articlekey=9246*

Neurotransmitters are manufactured, or **synthesized**, in our brains; many are made from amino acids that are in the foods we eat.

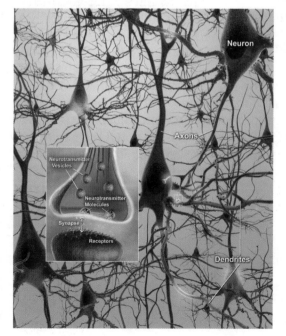

Neuron

Axons

Neurotransmitter Vesicles

Neurotransmitter Molecules

Synapse

Receptors

Dendrites

◀ **FIGURE 3.2**
A network of neurons and the transmission of electrical impulses by neurotransmitters. The large image shows the **axons**, which are, basically, the "senders" of the electrochemical impulses from one neuron to another, and the **dendrites**, which are the branches of a neuron that conduct the received message to the cell body of the (receiving) neuron. Synapses are located at various points on the dendrite branches. The inset shows a close-up of a synapse and the neurotransmitters moving across the synaptic gap. SOURCE: Image courtesy of the National Institute on Aging/National Institutes of Health.

In a process known as **reuptake**, the neurotransmitter is *reabsorbed* by the *presynaptic* neuron after the neurotransmitter has transmitted the neural impulse. Reuptake allows for recycling of the neurotransmitters and controls the level of chemical present in the synapse.

Although there are a number of different neurotransmitters, **serotonin**, **dopamine**, **epinephrine** (**adrenaline**), and **norepinephrine** are the neurotransmitters produced within our bodies that the tryptamine-based and phenethylamine-based psychedelics most closely resemble. Most psychedelic molecules are similarly structured to the molecules of the neurotransmitters that occur naturally in the brain.

20. What are agonists and antagonists?

Agonist molecules bind to receptors on a cell or neuron, provoking a process of change in the cell's functions. An **antagonist** inhibits these effects, and an **inverse agonist** results in effects opposite to those of the agonist. Certain synthetic psychotherapeutic medications are agonists and are used to mimic the effects of a natural (endogenous) compound, such as a neurotransmitter or hormone; other medications are antagonists and are prescribed to prevent or inhibit the neurotransmitters from binding to the receptors. Depending on the imbalance of the endogenous chemical—in other words, insufficient or excessive amounts of a particular neurotransmitter—synthetic psychotropic drugs are prescribed to correct the imbalance; frequently, an agonist–antagonist combination achieves the correct balance.

The term **endogenous** refers to a natural occurrence or state caused by elements within an organism or system; **exogenous** refers to factors that affect a system or organism from the outside. So, endogenous substances are those naturally occurring chemicals produced by our bodies within our bodies, such as the neurotransmitters mentioned previously. Exogenous substances are those that are "foreign" to our bodies, produced elsewhere but introduced into or administered to our systems. Many exogenous psychotherapeutic medicines are made to duplicate our endogenous neurotransmitters, and many psychoactive drugs that are endogenous in other forms of nature—the aforementioned plants, molds, fungi—are structurally similar to our naturally occurring neurotransmitters.

For example, the cause of Parkinson's disease is depletion of the endogenous neurotransmitter dopamine. Dopamine controls movement and motor functions and reward-motivated behavior; it performs a number of tasks in the autonomic nervous system as well, from releasing hormones to reducing insulin production. Dopamine can be made and administered intravenously, but it cannot reach the brain because of the **blood–brain barrier**.

DEFINITION
The blood–brain barrier is a highly selective permeable barrier that separates the circulating blood from the brain's extracellular fluid in the central nervous system.

L-DOPA is another naturally occurring chemical that can be manufactured, and it *does* cross the blood–brain barrier; it is a precursor to dopamine and its metabolic structure is very similar. When L-DOPA crosses into the central nervous system, it is converted to dopamine through interaction with an enzyme. L-DOPA is sold as a psychotropic drug that is used as medication for the Parkinson's patient to increase dopamine in their brains. Please see Figures 3.3(a) and Figure 3.3(b) for a comparison of

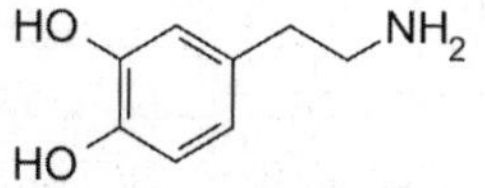

▲ FIGURE 3.3A
Diagram of the chemical structure of dopamine.

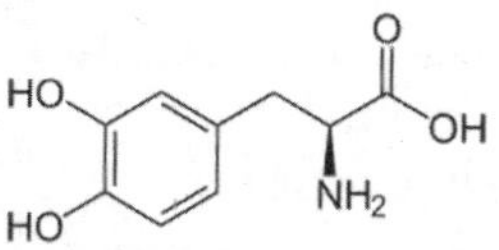

▲ FIGURE 3.3B
Diagram of the chemical structure of L-Dopa.

the chemical structures of the neurotransmitter dopamine and its "substitute," L-DOPA.

In this way, many psychedelic drugs "mimic" the chemical structures and effects of the naturally occurring—endogenous— chemicals in our brains. It is important to understand that many psychedelics are not too very unlike our own endogenous neurotransmitters, metabolically; it is reasonable to consider that if a manufactured medication that is a "substitute" for dopamine can help a Parkinson's patient, then research into how psychedelics could be manufactured to be medically beneficial as psychotherapeutic medications is a valid prospect.

22. What is the importance of serotonin?

Serotonin is the most well-known neurotransmitter. Its chemical name and structure is 5-hydroxytryptamine (5-HT) and, as the name suggests, it is a variant of tryptamine. Serotonin is the messenger of many basic brain and bodily functions. It controls moods such as depression, anxiety, pleasure, and contentment; it regulates sleep, appetite, and the movement of "smooth" muscles (muscles that move involuntarily, without our conscious thought, found in the walls of internal organs such as the stomach, intestine, and bladder) and blood vessels to regulate blood pressure and digestive functions. Self-esteem is linked to this neurotransmitter; depletion of serotonin can cause loss of self-image and self-esteem and, in turn, severe depression and self-destructive tendencies.

23. What is an entheogen?

The term **entheogen** literally means "generating the divine within." In the context of our purposes, an entheogen is a psychoactive substance that taps into the "God experience." The use of entheogens as sacraments in spiritual or religious ceremonies has been practiced since the dawn of spiritual awakening in mankind, and it is entirely plausible that these plants and fungi partaken by early man actually manifested the "other worldly" or spiritual consciousness that contributed to the birth of religions and the concept of an omniscient and omnipresent universal spirit or "God." That our ancestors ingested leaf, mushroom, mold, or cactus button and then experienced an opening of mind and a blossoming of a sense of connection to each other, as "we are all one and the universe holds us all in love," is a long- and well-accepted notion.

For many non-Western cultures, psychedelic drugs are considered spiritual tools or sacred medicine; they are entheogens. According to the article by Martin Ball (cited in the NOTE), today there are three officially recognized religions in the United States that

Many of the earliest human artifacts—from mushroom shaman effigies in prehistoric African cave paintings to marijuana incense burners in shrines in ancient Europe—depict entheogenic fungi and plants with clear associations to ritual and religious activity. The "foods of the gods" have been with us from the beginning.
— Martin Ball: *http://spiritualityhealth. com/articles/four-legal-entheogens-spiritual-explorer#sthash.6ptKttKl.dpuf*

legally use entheogens as sacraments in their ceremonies and religious practices. Members of the Native American Church consume peyote cactus buttons, and Santo Daime and Uniao do Vegetal drink a concoction known as ayahuasca, which is an infusion made from the *Banisteriopsis caapi* vine, in combination with other plants.

24. Are all psychedelic drugs entheogens?

An entheogen is really any substance or state that has spiritual properties. Psychedelics are distinguished as entheogens because the mind-altering properties, when the drugs are administered with careful attention paid to set and setting, create a sense of "oneness with the universe" and a spiritual uplifting. Dissociative hallucinations are not typical of the psychedelic experience, however, some entheogens (such as *Salvia divinorum*—a psychoactive plant that can induce "visions"—and ibogaine, which is a strong, long-lasting hallucinogen used traditionally in a coming-of-age ritual but also known for its modern use in treating opiate addiction) do produce dissociative hallucinations. The term entheogen encompasses the classical, well-known tryptamine-based psychedelics listed and described in Chapter 2, "Psychedelic Compounds," all of which are natural,

Entheogens show significant promise in psychotherapy and in treating OCD, cluster headaches, drug and alcohol addictions, and to help the terminally ill come to peace and acceptance with their life and death.

http://www.neurosoup.com/ entheogens-and-entactogens/

Entactogens' effects promote bonding between people, a stimulant effect, a sense of love and peace with the universe and all people, outstanding psychotherapeutic effects, happiness, and a sense of seeing the universe and all senses as they really are.

—Nicholas Novak, *NeuroSoup*, *http://www. neurosoup.com/entheogens-and-entactogens/*

provided by plant life and fungal sources. The health risks from most entheogenic substances are extremely low.

It is because they are entheogens that psychedelics show vast potential to be used as tools for psychotherapy. It is through the mind-expanding, consciousness-raising effects of the drugs that patients become self-aware, remember buried traumas, and become open to discussing themselves with their psychotherapists.

25. What are entactogens or empathogens?

Entactogens ("the touch within"), also called **empathogens**, are drugs whose effects are similar to entheogens but with less profoundly spiritual properties. Entactogens cause a feeling of bonding with other people—as the term "empathogen" suggests, these psychoactive drugs create a sense of empathy or an ability to identify with other people.

As a wrap-up to this chapter, a 20-minute video titled *God Is in the Neurons* is a fascinating exploration of the chemistry of the brain, its neurotransmitters, and neural connections to self-awareness, emotions, consciousness, and spirituality.

http://www.youtube.com/watch?v=oPEdDcs _8ZQ&feature=youtu.be

The most common empathogen is MDMA, or ecstasy, and the other phenethylamine-based psychoactives listed in Chapter 2 have empathogenic properties as well.

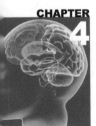

CHAPTER 4

How Do Psychoactive Medications Work in the Brain?

In Chapter 3 we learned some terms that concern the action of the neurons and chemicals in our brains. This chapter offers a brief recap of some of those terms and introduces a couple of new ones as we put together everything we've learned thus far and offer a rudimentary explanation of just what occurs when psychoactive substances enter our systems.

26. How important are the neurotransmitters?

In a word, crucial.

Because the neurotransmitter chemicals carry messages from one neuron to the other, they are the controlling factor of our thoughts, moods, movements, language, heartbeat, breathing . . . just everything about us. When the neurotransmitters are out of balance, unhealthy reactions can occur.

Neurotransmitter levels can be depleted in many ways. As a matter of fact, it is estimated that 86% of Americans have suboptimal neurotransmitter levels. Stress, poor diet, neurotoxins, genetic predisposition, drugs (prescription and recreational), alcohol, and caffeine usage can cause these levels to be out of optimal range.

—The Brain Wellness Program, *www.neurogistics.com*

Remember that neurotransmitters are endogenous chemicals; our bodies manufacture them. Our bodies need them. Recall also our discussion of dopamine and Parkinson's disease—if an imbalance occurs, it's not always a simple matter of just popping a pill of the particular chemical that needs to be repleted or depleted; frequently other chemicals are needed to assist.

27. How do psychoactive chemicals interact with the neurotransmitters?

If neurotransmitters transmit communications between neurons or between neurons and other cells, we can think of psychoactive compounds as interrupting or altering those communications, and psychoactive drugs can do that in several different ways in their roles as agonists or antagonists (recall the definitions of agonist and antagonist from Chapter 3):

- They can become **precursors**, which are substances from which other substances are formed, especially by natural processes. Such was the case of L-DOPA in our Parkinson's example in Chapter 3.
- They can inhibit the natural manufacture, known as **synthesis**, of the neurotransmitter. Many neurotransmitters

are synthesized from amino acids in the foods we eat. If our bodies are synthesizing too much of a particular neurotransmitter, an effective drug can slow down the manufacture.

- They can prevent the presynaptic vesicles from storing the neurotransmitter. Recall that the vesicles are little storage bins for the neurotransmitters, located beneath the membrane on the presynaptic neuron.
- They can interfere with the release of the neurotransmitter by stimulating or inhibiting the action.
- They can alter the receiving of the transmission by stimulating or blocking postsynaptic receptors.
- They can stimulate the **autoreceptors**, inhibiting neurotransmitter release. The autoreceptor is a receptor located on the *pre*synaptic neuron. It might help to think of it as a "feedback" mechanism. When the neurotransmitter is released, the autoreceptor recognizes the action and will function to control internal cell processes, inhibiting either further release or ongoing synthesis of the neurotransmitter.
- They can also, however, *block* autoreceptors, which increases neurotransmitter release or hastens its manufacture.
- They can inhibit neurotransmission breakdown.
- They can block the neurotransmitter reuptake (reabsorption) process by the presynaptic neuron.

There is a great deal going on with these processes, as you can see; imbalances in the makeup of the system, or deviations in the metabolic pathway of the chemicals can be further confused or controlled by exogenous psychoactive compounds. Recall from Chapter 2: the appropriate psychotropic drugs—those psychoactives that are prescribed—are usually agonists or antagonists; they can effectively balance the amount of neurotransmitter that successfully binds to the receptor; conversely, the wrong drug—or even the correct drug but in an incorrect dosage—can further disrupt the process.

28. How do psychedelics work in the brain?

Recall that psychedelics are psychoactive drugs; the processes through which they affect the neurotransmitters are the same as those described in the answer to the previous question. They can act as agonists or antagonists and alter the balance of neurotransmitters. Recall also that many psychedelics are metabolically very similar to our endogenous chemicals. However, even understanding this, the exact action of the psychedelics is poorly understood. It is thought by many researchers that psychedelics work by inhibiting the brain's natural tendency to block perceptions; in other words, in normal consciousness, our brains pick and choose that which we wish to perceive. When a psychedelic is introduced, it prevents the brain from being selective. and allows myriad perceptions to be recognized.

As Aldous Huxley wrote in *The Doors of Perception,*

> The function of the brain and nervous system is to protect us from being overwhelmed and confused by this mass of largely useless and irrelevant knowledge, by shutting out most of what we should otherwise perceive or remember at any moment, and leaving only that very small and special selection which is likely to be practically useful.

Huxley further believed that, under the influence of mescaline or LSD, this mechanism is switched off, and we are treated to an overwhelming confusion of sights, sounds, colors, and feelings—all of which are actually present, but we normally do not get a chance to experience them. This theory is what is meant when psychedelics are described as "expanding" our minds and opening up our conscious awareness. Huxley was not a neuroscientist, but contemporary studies demonstrate that, in some respects, he was not far off the mark.

Another theory is that psychedelics put our brains into a "shut down" state, and instead of perceiving what is "out there," the brain focuses on internal imagery—the stuff of memories and dreams. The idea that this class of drugs, by encouraging the brain to shut out external "noise" and focus on the internal self, memories, and imagination, supports the consideration that psychedelics could be useful and valid tools for psychotherapy.

It is hoped that further research will unveil the "magic" of the way psychedelics work, how the brain operates and, crucially, how we can develop medical treatments to help us use this information to improve the lives of patients whose struggle to manage their emotional memories is the cause of their suffering.

How Do Psychedelic Drugs Work in the Brain? is an informative video by Dr. Robin Carhart-Harris, one of today's leading researchers at the Imperial College in London. Dr. Carhart-Harris, in quite understandable fashion, talks about his scientific research and brain imaging work involving psilocybin and the effects and potential therapeutic uses of psychedelic drugs.

ON THE WEB

http://www.youtube.com/ watch?v=jT5dZDnJ6J4

29. Why are psychedelics not being used as medicines?

This is an excellent question; it does seem that the potential benefit of these drugs is such that they would be unusually helpful psychotherapeutically. The fact is that research on these drugs has been stalled for the last 30–40 years because the drugs are illegal. In the meantime, psychopharmacology has developed any number (and a continually growing number) of synthetic psychopharmaceuticals to treat a variety of psychiatric illnesses (as discussed in Chapter 1). Many of these pharmaceuticals have serious side effects, particularly the antidepressants and antipsychotics. Testament to this is any television commercial advertising a drug—the list of dangers and side effects often sounds quite alarming. There will be more detail and comparisons with the psychedelics in later chapters.

The next few chapters will concern the history of research efforts into the use of psychedelics and will offer an explanation of why research has been halted.

ON THE WEB

Part 2 of *Psychedelic Drugs– The Unexplained* focuses on the reasons for the unfortunate hiatus in psychedelic research. *http://www.youtube.com/ watch?v=rH5MQYdae5Y*

PART TWO

A Brief History
of Research Efforts

In these chapters, we offer a brief history of psychedelic research. We discuss research in the early years of the 20th century and introduce pioneers of psychedelic research and their contributions to studies done in the mid-1900s. Chapter 7 offers explanations for the lack of research in the latter half of the 20th century.

A Brief History: From Ages Past to Research in the Early 20th Century

Historically, there have been three great eras of research into psychedelic culture and science. The first began a couple of decades before the dawn of the twentieth century; the second, and generally the most well-known, was the "flower-power" era of the 1960s; and the third, excitingly, is the one we are in right now.

30. When were psychedelics first discovered?

As mentioned previously, psychedelic entheogens have been used since the beginning of the existence of mankind and have spawned various religious and spiritual practices. For millennia, sacred plants have been an essential tool for altering consciousness. There is robust anthropological and archaeological evidence that hosts of plants and fungi were used in a shamanistic context for at least 5,000 years—since the very earliest written records.

Figure 5.1 shows four "mushroom stones" dating from 1000 B.C. to 500 A.D. The spiritual significance of the stones was probably of great consequence, given that each of the figures shown is approximately a foot tall.

Ancient paintings of mushroom-ed humanoids dating to 5,000 B.C. have been found in caves on the Tassili plateau of Northern Algeria.
NOTE
Central and Southern America cultures built temples to mushroom gods and carved "mushroom stones." These stone carvings in the shape of mushrooms, or in which figures are depicted under the cap of a mushroom, have been dated to as early as 1000 B.C.–500 B.C.

—http://www.erowid.org/plants/mushrooms/mushrooms_history.shtml

Recorded evidence suggests that our ancient ancestors preserved their psychedelic mushrooms by storing them in honey, and that the Aztecs served them with honey or chocolate at some of their spiritual ceremonies. The Aztecs used a variety of entheogenic plants: peyote, morning glory seeds, *Salvia divinorum*, and Jimson weed (Datura), among others lesser known.

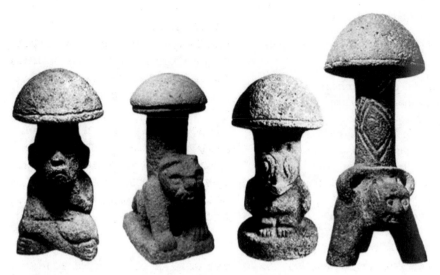

▲ FIGURE 5.1
Four mushroom stones dating from 1000 B.C. to 500 A.D.

31. Were these plants and fungi used only in ceremonies?

Some of these plants, roots, fungi, and molds have also been used as medications for centuries.

An essential feature of shamanistic belief is that it is a method of communication between the human and the spiritual world; there is almost always a "calling on the gods" for healings and a medicinal purpose to the methods and practice. Shamans have always been considered to be skilled as herbalists, botanists, anatomists, and physicians, as well as psychiatrists and priests, and it is highly likely that both psychoactive and nonpsychoactive plants and herbs have been—and still are—used in shamanistic healings.

Ergot (*Claviceps purpurea*), is a fungus that grows on rye and other grasses and crops; it contains lysergic acid, which is a major component of LSD. It is known to have vasoconstrictive (constriction of a blood vessel) properties, and, for

In 2005, researchers used radiocarbon dating and alkaloid analysis to study two specimens of peyote buttons found in archaeological digs from a site called Shumla Cave No. 5 on the Rio Grande in Texas. The results dated the specimens to between 3780 and 3660 B.C. . . . This indicates that native North Americans were likely to have used peyote since at least five and a half thousand years ago.

http://en.wikipedia.org/wiki/Peyote.

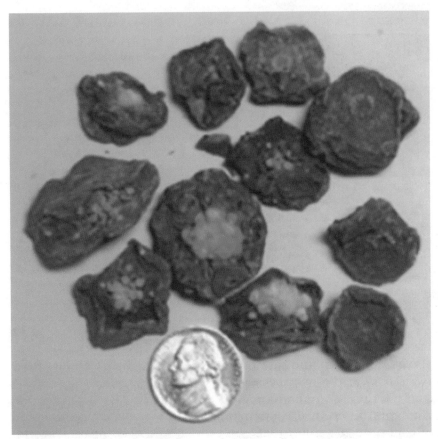

▲ FIGURE 5.2
Dried peyote buttons, approximately the size of a nickel.

hundreds of years, it was used to induce contractions and to stem after-childbirth hemorrhaging.

32. When did psychedelics first come to the attention of the scientific community?

In our more recent history, psychedelics were "rediscovered" and became of interest to the medical community between the 1880s and the 1920s, particularly with regard to the mescaline of the peyote cactus and hashish (opium received a great deal of attention during this period as well; however, opium is *not* a psychedelic; opium is a narcotic, which dulls the senses and is addictive; it is not the focus of this book).

In 1886, Dr. John Raleigh Briggs of Dallas, Texas, ingested part of a peyote button and a year later published a short article on his experience. Though the cactus had received mention in botanical studies since as early as the 1840s, Briggs's article appears to be the first written description of the psychological and physical effects caused by ingesting the cactus. Briggs's personal account came to the attention of the Parke-Davis pharmaceutical company in Detroit, Michigan, and became the impetus for several years of intense research on the psychological and therapeutic effects of the cactus plant.

NOTE

According to the National Institute on Drug Abuse, "The use of cannabis for purposes of healing predates recorded history. The earliest written reference is found in the 15th-century B.C. Chinese Pharmacopeia, the Rh-Ya" (NIDA, *Marijuana Research Findings*, 1976, 1977).

PRACTICAL TIP

There is such a great deal of information about the history of the medicinal use of cannabis through the ages that it is impossible to include it all in these pages. We urge readers to visit a quite thorough and well-substantiated timeline of medical cannabis use from 2900 B.C. to the present:

http://medicalmarijuana.procon.org/ view.timeline.php?timelineID=000026

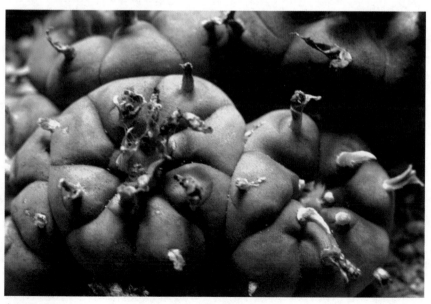

▲ FIGURE 5.3
Living peyote cactus.

33. Who performed some of this earliest research and what did it entail?

After being in contact with Dr. Briggs, Parke-Davis, in addition to performing their own analyses, distributed samples of the peyote buttons to pharmacologists; among them was Louis Lewin, the German pharmacologist whom we introduced in Chapter 2. Lewin's focus of study was the mind-altering effects and the pharmacological makeup of various plants. Lewin also developed a classification system based on the effects of the plants he studied. In 1887, Lewin published the first detailed analysis of the peyote cactus, and a variety of the cactus was named *Anhalonium lewinii* in his honor.

In 1896, almost a decade after Lewin's report on the peyote cactus, American neurologist and novelist S. Weir Mitchell wrote the first Western medical report describing the cactus and the psychological effects of mescaline on humans, "The Effects of Anhelonium Lewinii (the Mescal Button)," for the *British Medical Journal*. His paper was followed a year later by two articles from the British physician and psychologist Henry Havelock Ellis: "The Phenomena of Mescal Intoxication," in 1897, and "Mescal: A New Artificial Paradise." Ellis and Mitchell were keen proponents of the mescaline experience and their works inspired many others to explore the sensory and spiritual delights of the plant.

Another major breakthrough occurred in 1897 when German pharmacologist Arthur Carl Wilhelm Heffter succeeded in isolating mescaline from the peyote cactus, which was the first time a naturally occurring psychedelic had been identified and extracted in this way. At the end of the nineteenth century, mescaline was the only widely known psychedelic drug in existence.

34. When was LSD discovered?

Albert Hofmann was a research chemist working in the 1930s at Sandoz Laboratories in Switzerland as a member of a team of pre-war chemists and psychopharmacologists. His main area of research involved the synthesis of various preparations based on ergot because of its vasoconstrictive properties (described in Question 31). The discovery of LSD (lysergic acid diethylamide) was an offshoot of Hofmann's work with ergot; lysergic acid is a naturally occurring compound produced by the fungus. The psychoactive qualities of ergot are recognized as having been responsible for outbreaks of St. Anthony's Fire in the Middle Ages; these were peculiar epidemics of mass psychosis, hysteria, and death when entire communities became poisoned by bread made from moldy flour. It is debated whether ergot was the source of "bewitchments" that spurred the Salem witch trials. In 1938, Hofmann produced the 25th in his series of synthesized combinations of chemicals based around the structure of lysergic acid: lysergic acid diethylamide, which he called LSD-25 (the "S" in the acronym stands for *saure*, the German word for acid). It is widely believed that this moment in 1938 was the first time LSD was brought into existence.

35. Is it true that Hofmann's discovery of LSD was accidental?

Before discovering its psychoactive properties, Hofmann put aside his research of LSD-25 and did not return to it again until 1943, when he synthesized a fresh batch. It was during this process that Hofmann accidentally absorbed through the skin a small quantity of the drug and experienced a peculiar psychological episode characterized by dizziness and altered perceptions.

> *I became affected by a remarkable restlessness, combined with a slight dizziness. At home I lay down and sank into a not unpleasant intoxicated-like condition, characterized by an extremely stimulated imagination. In a dreamlike state, with eyes closed (I found the daylight to be unpleasantly glaring), I perceived an uninterrupted stream of fantastic pictures, extraordinary shapes with intense, kaleidoscopic play of colors. After some two hours this condition faded away.*
>
> —Albert Hofmann, *LSD: My Problem Child: Reflections on Sacred Drugs, Mysticism and Science*

Three days later, April 19, 1943, convinced that the LSD-25 must contain significant and unusual properties if effects could be felt after absorbing a minute amount, Hofmann began a series of self-experiments and purposely ingested a 0.25-mg quantity of the drug, which he assumed to be a small dose, but he soon realized he had underestimated the potency of his discovery.

His bicycle ride home from the laboratory is a now-famous story of the first "acid trip" taken by a human being.

". . . little by little I could begin to enjoy the unprecedented colors and plays of shapes that persisted behind my closed eyes. Kaleidoscopic, fantastic images surged in on me, alternating, variegated, opening and then closing themselves in circles and spirals, exploding in colored fountains, rearranging and hybridizing themselves in constant flux. . ."

—Albert Hofmann, *LSD: My Problem Child: Reflections on Sacred Drugs, Mysticism and Science.*

After this experience, Hofmann realized that he had made a remarkable discovery. Here was a drug with immeasurable

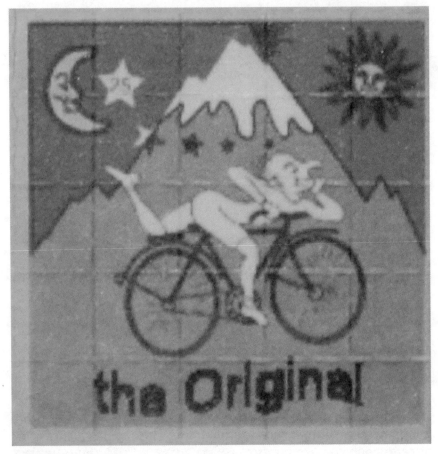

▲ **FIGURE 5.4**
25 squares of LSD blotter paper showing the complete pattern that depicts Hofmann's Bicycle Day.
SOURCE: Courtesy YttriumOx.

potential, powerfully active even in the most miniscule of doses (it is still recognized today as the most potent psychoactive substance known to science, by an order of magnitude far beyond any other known compounds), and Hofmann believed that LSD could be beneficial for use in psychotherapy because of its "intense and introspective nature."

36. When did LSD become available for use in psychotherapy?

After a few years of Phase 1 investigation of the drug by staff at the Sandoz laboratories, testing it on animals to evaluate its degree of toxicity and potential safety for human consumption, in 1947, Werner Stoll, a colleague of Hofmann, published the first academic description of the mental effects of LSD on humans.

The laboratory studies concluded that despite the drug's intense mental effects, LSD was not considered to be physiologically toxic and was deemed safe for human consumption. Hofmann was eager to share LSD with any respectable psychiatrist who might be able to develop useful research utilizing the new compound and, at the end of the first half of the 20th century, began distribution of the drug, under the brand name *Delysid*, to psychiatrists worldwide.

In this chapter we have covered the earliest use and research of psychedelic compounds. Our next chapters describe events of the second half of the 20th century.

Psychedelic Research and Pioneers in the mid-1900s

CHAPTER
6

The beginning of the second half of the twentieth century held exciting promise for the psychiatric community. The discovery, research, and dissemination of LSD-25 by Hofmann and Stoll at the Sandoz laboratories spurred many new approaches to research into the processes of mental illness. Modern psychoanalysis, or "talk therapy," the merits and manners of which were still being debated, was becoming a more established and accepted form of treatment, growing from the work of Freud and

Jung and their colleagues in the earlier decades of the century. And now! Here were the recent discoveries of the synthesized mescaline and LSD compounds to open the unconscious part of the brain and potentially benefit efforts to develop increasingly effective methods of psychoanalysis.

The future may teach us how to exercise a direct influence, by means of particular chemical substances, upon . . . the neural apparatus. It may be that there are other still undreamt of possibilities of therapy.

—Sigmund Freud

37. Were psychedelics being used to treat mental illnesses at this time?

In 1949, an article by psychiatrists at the Boston Psychopathic Hospital (now the Massachusetts Mental Health Center) in the United States was the first published study to describe the use of LSD in treating psychiatric patients. In these earliest recorded studies, LSD was used as a psychotomimetic (recall from Chapter 2, the meaning of psychotomimetic is "to mimic psychoses"); however, it was not used to treat patients in these studies; it was for doctors and other clinicians to take themselves and to administer to control subjects in order to glimpse what it feels like to have schizophrenia. The remarkable psychological qualities of LSD, coupled with the fact that it was from a known organic agent, excited many researchers; here was a way to understand how schizophrenia works at the brain level.

In 1950, Anthony Busch and Warren Johnson of St. Louis, Missouri, USA, published the results of a study describing the effects of LSD when given at low doses (maximum 40 mcg) to 29 patients; most were suffering from paranoid schizophrenia or mania. Busch and Johnson concluded that the drug appeared to improve access to the patients' otherwise inaccessible mental states and proposed further studies to consider whether the drug could have a beneficial role in the practice of psychotherapy.

LSD Experiment—"Schizophrenic Model Psychosis induced by LSD-25" was filmed in 1955; it shows an experiment on a human subject. The introductory footage explains that experiments were made using LSD to induce "artificial insanity" in order to prove that the mentally ill were not "inhabited by the devil."

http://www.youtube.com/watch?v=M7fOuPTZtWI

38. What was the MK-Ultra program?

There has been much written about the experimentation with psychoactive substances by government military agencies in America and Europe. In the 1950s, the CIA had a low-profile project called MK-Ultra, a research operation into human mind control. Slipping drugs (especially LSD) and other chemicals to unsuspecting individuals was one method, among others (hypnosis, sensory deprivation, isolation, verbal and sexual abuse, torture), employed in experiments in order to study unwitting human subjects' reactions and their altered mental states. The "top secret" project achieved notoriety when many horror stories and complaints subsequently emerged with regard to these covert and unethical activities; the discreditable MK-Ultra program was shut down—but not until 1973. There will be more details about this program in later pages.

39. Who were some of the notable clinicians and researchers in the early part of this era?

British psychiatrists Ronald Sandison and Humphry Osmond, researcher Stanislav Grof from Czechoslovakia, and research psychologist Timothy Leary (with colleague Richard Alpert) of the United States were the most notably significant proponents of psychedelic research. Other names, such as Aldous Huxley, "Cappy" Al Hubbard, Abbie Hoffman, Allen Ginsberg, and others are inextricably associated with the time, as well, although they were not technicians, analysts, or scientists. There are brief synopses of some of their stories in the following pages; for more detailed accounts of their research and for their biographies, the reader is urged to follow the web links to videos and online information and to read suggested published books and articles.

40. What was Dr. Humphry Osmond's major contribution to the field?

"To fathom hell or fly angelic,
Just take a pinch of psychedelic."

—Humphry Osmond in a letter to Aldous Huxley

Through his research efforts, Dr. Humphry Osmond (1917–2004) was among the first in his field to come to recognize the possible value of psychedelics for psychiatric therapy and personal growth. Learning about the studies being conducted in the United States into the possibility that LSD could be used as a psychotomimetic and that the drug could possibly reveal some understanding of schizophrenia, Osmond and his friend and colleague Dr. John Smythies researched the effects of mescaline on patients who were diagnosed with schizophrenia at the Weyburn Mental Hospital in Saskatchewan, Canada.

Osmond conducted a number of important psychedelic drug trials throughout the 1950s in collaboration with Dr. Abram Hoffer, Canadian biochemist and psychiatrist (Hoffer later became internationally recognized for his research into the use of vitamins and nutrients to treat mental disorders and for his work with addiction therapy). Osmond and Hoffer gained particular attention for studies using LSD to treat patients with **alcohol dependency syndrome**. At the time, there was a prevailing theory that the delirium tremens (DTs) are so terrifying for alcoholics that a psychosis is created when an alcoholic "hits bottom," which leads effectively to sobriety in many cases. Osborn and Hoffer attempted to create DT-like experiences by administering psychedelics to their patients. The initial theory was disproved because the LSD experiences did not frighten patients in quite the way the researchers had imagined; many of their patients actually enjoyed the mind-altering effects they felt after ingesting the drug. However, and more importantly, the outcome of the experiments did lead patients to successful recovery from alcohol dependence; this success was attributed to the entheogenic effects of the drug and a conviction that when a patient has had an experience as profound as the spiritual awakening brought about by LSD, the effects of alcohol pale in comparison. Most patients did not even have to struggle to conquer a desire for alcohol after the LSD-associated therapy.

Worthy of mention is that Bill Wilson, cofounder of Alcoholics Anonymous (AA) took LSD under Osmond's supervision in the 1950s, the first occasion being on August 29, 1956. *Pass It On*, Wilson's official AA biography, states, "Bill was enthusiastic about his [LSD] experience; he felt it helped him eliminate many barriers erected by the self, or ego, that stand in the way of one's direct experience of the cosmos and of God." (*http://mywordlikefire.com/tag/grace/*)

Because the AA approach to sobriety is through surrender to a sense of spirituality, and LSD is a powerful entheogen, Wilson believed that LSD, administered in a controlled clinical setting, could play a potential role in the treatment of addiction.

It is a generally acknowledged fact in spiritual development that ego reduction makes the influx of God's grace possible. If, therefore, under LSD we can have a temporary reduction, so that we can better see what we are and where we are going—well, that might be of some help. The goal might become clearer. So I consider LSD to be of some value to some people, and practically no damage to anyone.

—Bill Wilson, *Pass It On* (p. 370); *http://mywordlikefire.com/tag/grace/*

Osmond and colleagues fine-tuned the process further, adding elements of supportive psychotherapy and, before long, were able to boast of abstinence rates of 50%–90%, which far surpasses all other treatments for alcohol addiction before or since. However, experimental protocols were less rigorous in the '50s than they are today; there has been some criticism of Osmond and Hoffer's trials, with accusations that the experiments lacked adequate controls.

Osmond is also known for having introduced author and intellectual Aldous Huxley (1894–1963) to mescaline, Huxley's first psychedelic experience. As mentioned in Chapter 2, a correspondence between Osmond and Huxley led to the term "psychedelic," which gained popular usage once Osmond introduced the word at a conference in 1957.

41. Why was Aldous Huxley's involvement with psychedelics significant?

The theories and writings of Aldous Huxley contributed significantly to the advancement of the use of psychedelics because of his reputation as one of the foremost philosophers and deep thinkers of his time. Huxley dedicated much of his life to his pursuit of knowledge and enlightenment. His thought-provoking novels, philosophical works, essays, and poems examined ideals, humanities, ethics, and the use of biotechnology and

ON THE WEB

For more details on Osmond's research and current research on psychedelic therapy for alcohol addiction, you might enjoy a brief lecture by Michael Bogenschutz, MD: "Psilocybin-Assisted Treatment for Alcohol Dependence." *http://www.maps.org/conference/ps13michaelbogenschutz/*

There is a short film, which was recorded in 1955, of a famous experiment in which Humphry Osmond administered mescaline to British parliament member Christopher Mayhew. The film gained notoriety because, ironically, it was *not* shown at the time! It was intended to be broadcast on the BBC, however, it was shelved because a committee of psychiatrists deemed that it was not an authentic "mystical" experience, although Mayhew himself maintains that it was. *https://www.youtube.com/watch?v=Eh8IBLs61_M*

psychopharmacology in futuristic societies to create utopian vs. dystopian ("negative" utopia) worlds, among other topics.

In 1953, Aldous Huxley, although not a psychotherapy patient, contacted Dr. Humphry Osmond and volunteered to participate in experiments with mescaline that Osmond was conducting. Osmond first gave mescaline to Huxley in May of 1953; Huxley was almost 60 years old.

After Huxley's experiences with mescaline, he advocated the use of psychedelic drugs to assist in achieving clarity of perception, self-knowledge, and understanding of the interconnectedness of the universe. Huxley, whose later literary works explore levels of consciousness, mysticism, Universality, and enlightenment, theorized that there is a "door" in the brain that can be opened in order to enter a higher realm of consciousness.

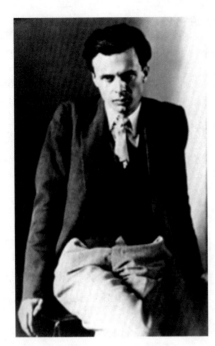

▲ **FIGURE 6.1**
Aldous Huxley.

By the end of his life, Huxley was considered, in some academic circles, a leader of modern thought and an intellectual of the highest rank.

NOTE

http://www.goodreads.com/author/show/3487.Aldous_Huxley

There is a brief video about Huxley and Osmond that describes Huxley's theories and his mescaline experience.

ON THE WEB

http://www.youtube.com/watch?v=mbI4f1WvN9w

42. When did Huxley first try LSD?

Through Dr. Osmond, Huxley was introduced to "Captain Trips," Alfred Hubbard, who gave Huxley his first taste of LSD on December 24, 1955.

"What came through the closed door," Huxley stated, "was the realization—not the knowledge, for this wasn't verbal or abstract—but the direct, total awareness, from the inside, so to say, of Love as the primary and fundamental cosmic fact."

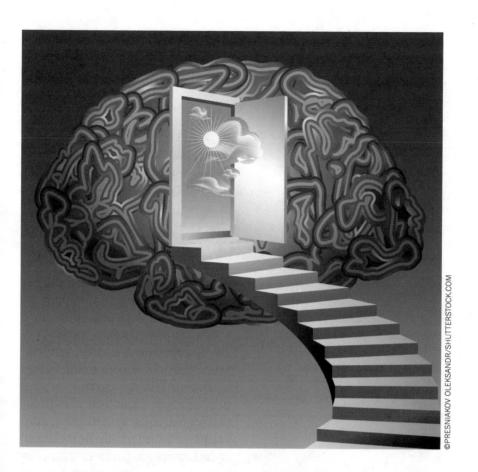

©PRESNIAKOV OLEKSANDR/SHUTTERSTOCK.COM

Huxley spent the remainder of his life deeply involved with the psychedelic culture and considered Hubbard and Osmond to be his mentors.

PRACTICAL TIP

The Huxley quote appears in *Acid Dreams: The Complete Social History of LSD: The CIA, The Sixties, and Beyond* by Martin A. Lee and Bruce Shalin, pages of which are available at *http://www.levity.com/ aciddreams/samples/capthubbard.html*

43. Why was Alfred Hubbard called "Captain Trips"?

Alfred Hubbard (1901–1982), had several nicknames—and wore many different "hats." During the '50s and '60s, "Cappy," as he was called by his friends, also became known as the "Johnny Appleseed of LSD" and "Captain Trips" because he flagrantly and prodigiously shared LSD with as many people as he could. Traveling the world with a leather bag that held a cornucopia of LSD-25, mescaline, and psilocybin, Hubbard introduced

NOTE

PRACTICAL TIP

thousands of people to psychedelics: psychiatrists, physicians, researchers, church leaders, fellow spies, politicians, and government officials.

Hubbard was quite a colorful character; part humanitarian, part businessman, part therapist, with a cloak-and-dagger life style. Though there is not much written about him, he was probably one of the most influential proponents of psychedelic drug research and use of that time in that, with his high-level government and business contacts, he was able to procure and widely distribute synthesized psychedelics. He believed that psychedelics would be a boon to mankind and could alter the belief systems of the world populations to embrace universal peace and love.

44. What research efforts were going on in the UK?

You may recall from Chapter 2 that it was Dr. Ronald Sandison (1916–2010) who coined the term "psycholytic" for these synthesized compounds; he and other physicians in the UK had a very different approach to LSD than did researchers in America. In the UK, there was not much agreement that LSD could be a psychotomimetic; psychiatrists in the UK and continental Europe believed that the nature and quality of the experience was not at all like schizophrenia. Unlike suffering from continually present, unmanageable delusions that are symptomatic of psychoses, on LSD one is aware that he or she has taken a drug and knows that in a few hours the experience will subside. Consequently, few psychiatrists in Britain thought LSD helped them to understand schizophrenia.

Sandison used LSD as part of his psychotherapy program at Powick Hospital in Gloucestershire in the United Kingdom. He administered the drug to patients who, unable to face their deep-seated traumas, did not respond to traditional psychotherapeutic drugs or methods because they had repressed the associated memories and fears from their conscious minds. Sandison found that, in the clinical setting, the effects of LSD created a nonordinary state of consciousness that encouraged patients to unlock their distressful, repressed memories, allowing psychoanalysis with their doctors to more effectively work through the traumas that caused their debilitating neuroses and anxieties. Furthermore, the entheogenic qualities of the drug allowed patients to feel a sense of spiritual growth, insight, and self-understanding.

 Transpersonal has been defined as "experiences in which the sense of identity or self extends beyond (trans) the individual or personal to encompass wider aspects of humankind, life, psyche or cosmos."

—*http://en.wikipedia.org/wiki/ Transpersonal_psychology*

The *Journal of Transpersonal Psychology* defines transpersonal psychology as being "concerned with the study of humanity's highest potential, and with the recognition, understanding, and realization of unitive, spiritual, and transcendent states of consciousness."

In 1954, Dr. Sandison published a paper describing a series of 36 cases of LSD-assisted psychotherapy patients, "The Therapeutic Value of Lysergic Acid Diethylamide in Mental Illness," in *The Journal of Mental Science* (now the *British Journal of Psychiatry*), which described how, by using LSD, he was able to reawaken a therapeutic response from patients who had been experiencing treatment resistance. Also in 1954, Sandison built a special-purpose LSD clinic to treat patients who had been failing to make progress under "normal" psychotherapy; it was the earliest center for large-scale psychotherapeutic use of LSD, and over the next decade Sandison and colleagues used LSD in treatment of thousands of patients whose previous therapy had failed.

In 1954, there seemed to be promise of great advancement in the world of psychiatry and the therapeutic use of psychedelic compounds.

45. Were psychedelics being used in Europe?

In Europe, psychedelic research was taking off. Stanislav Grof (1931–) began observing LSD psychotherapy sessions in 1954 when he was a medical student at Charles University in Prague, and the experience influenced his decision to direct his career to the study of nonordinary states of consciousness. He is one of the founders of **transpersonal psychology**, which is often referred to as "spiritual psychology."

ON THE WEB

A two-part video, "Stan Grof About His LSD Experience and Research," is quite interesting:

Part 1: http://www.youtube.com/watch?v=5ig3eU_oDS0

Part 2: http://www.youtube.com/watch?v=-tSRHStwOPU

PRACTICAL TIP

Dr. Grof also has two websites that offer more detailed information and videos about his work and his philosophies:

www.stanislavgrof.com/ and *www.holotropic.com/*

In contrast to Sandison's **psycholytic method**, which prescribed low-to-medium doses of LSD in repeated sessions, Dr. Grof (who moved to the United States in 1967 to work at Johns Hopkins University) and researchers in the United States tended to follow a single—or infrequent—high-dose session (up to 500 micrograms of LSD) with subsequent *non*drug sessions of psychotherapy, during which the experiences and sensations that were revealed in the drug session were explored and analyzed. This method came to be called **psychedelic psychotherapy**.

Dr. Grof has been a pioneering researcher in this area, studying both psychedelic drug-induced and nondrug-induced nonordinary states of consciousness; he has developed a highly systemized theory describing how early prenatal and birth experiences can be reexperienced when in nonordinary states of consciousness.

Stanislav Grof is unique among the researchers discussed in this chapter because his work spans the mid-20th century to the current day. He remains actively involved with psychedelic research, and you will meet him again in later chapters.

46. Did Timothy Leary make any valid contribution in terms of research?

"Timothy Leary was without question one of the most controversial figures of his era, if not the 20th century. He was a polarizing figure in a time of generational conflict, a bold challenger of the status quo"

—http://timothyleary.org/#1

Of the researchers mentioned, readers are probably most familiar with the name Timothy Leary (1920–1996) and his well-known slogans, "Turn On, Tune In, Drop Out"; "Think for Yourself"; "Question Authority." Leary is identified with the "hippie" culture, "flower power," "make love, not war," "give peace a chance" days of the 1960s. The fact that Dr. Leary was a knowledgeable research psychologist before he arrived at Harvard in 1959 is often overlooked, and the abuse of the psychedelic medium among students and the general public in the late '60s is often attributed to him, although it is more likely that the yoke of blame rests across several shoulders. Leary authored 30 books and nearly 400 research papers, essays, and articles, and he interacted with many of the leading intellectuals, writers, musicians, and artists of the time.

Leary's main area of psychological research was in developing methods of measuring human personality characteristics and determining patterns of interpersonal processes, which could then be used to diagnose mental disorders.

47. How did Leary become involved with psychedelics?

Leary's research into the human personality led him to become intrigued with the hows and whys of the **transformation of behavioral characteristics.** In 1957, there appeared in *Life* magazine an article by mycologist (mycology is the study of mushrooms) Gordon Wasson, which became the first wide-scale mention of psychedelic drugs to occur in contemporary Western consciousness. The article led to wide interest in the subject and captured Leary's attention. Leary traveled to Mexico in 1960 with the intention of trying *Psilocybe mexicana* mushrooms; this was his first experience with mind-altering drugs (other than alcohol), and the event convinced Leary that the mushroom had positive transformative powers and could alter an individual's personality and spiritual direction; on his return to Harvard, he decided to dedicate his research to the still relatively new developments in the use of psychedelic drugs in psychiatric therapy. After the mushroom trip Leary commented,

"I learned more about my brain and its possibilities in the five hours after taking these mushrooms than I had in the preceding fifteen years of studying and doing research in psychology."

Together with colleague Richard Alpert (now known as Ram Dass), Leary set up and ran the **Harvard Psilocybin Project,** which included a course of experiments at the Concord Prison in Concord, Massachusetts, and the now-famous Marsh Chapel experiment in Boston.

48. What was the Concord Prison study?

The Concord Prison study involved 36 prisoners (some sources say 32 prisoners) who were given synthetic psilocybin combined with guided psychotherapy. Leary and Alpert and associates' intent was to evaluate the effects of the mushroom on the rehabilitation of released prisoners. They hoped that the study would demonstrate that psilocybin therapy could lower criminal recidivism rates. After the psilocybin therapy by Leary and his associates, the recidivism rate for those involved in the Concord Prison experiments dropped to 20%, compared to the 60% statistic for the general, nationwide prison population. The experimenters concluded that psilocybin-assisted group psychotherapy (inside the prison), together with a follow-up, post-release support program modeled on Alcoholics Anonymous, could bring about long-term reduction in overall criminal recidivism rates, though Leary himself admitted that the results were "extremely tentative."

49. Why is the Marsh Chapel experiment "famous"?

The Marsh Chapel experiment, also known as "the Good Friday experiment," was a PhD project conceived by Walter N. Pahnke (1931–1971), a graduate student in theology at Harvard Divinity School, under Leary's supervision. Pahnke was investigating whether psilocybin could induce a spiritual-type experience in students of theology—people who were already predisposed toward concepts of a religious nature. The subjects were from the Andover Newton Theological Seminary and the Harvard Divinity School and other Boston-area theological schools. The study stands out as being famous—partly because it was conducted on Good Friday, 1962, at Boston University's Marsh Chapel (shown in Figure 6.3), partly because Leary was involved, and partly because it was one of the most thoroughly designed **double-blind, placebo-controlled** psychedelic studies of its day. Most psychedelic studies of the time produced little more than anecdotal data; the Marsh Chapel experiment was scientifically measured and documented. Furthermore, the experiment, ever since, has been debated with regard to the extent of proving the entheogenic capabilities of psilocybin and, hence, other psychedelic compounds.

In order to study whether the drug actually created mystical experiences, a structured set of criteria (originally designed by W. T. Stace, professor of philosophy at Princeton University,

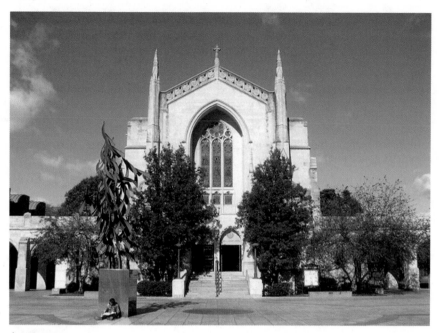

▲ FIGURE 6.2
Marsh Chapel, Boston University; site of the Good Friday experiment in 1962. Boston University Marsh Chapel, Boston MA by John Phelan (own work). Licensed under Creative Commons Attribution 3.0 via Wikimedia Commons.

to characterize a true, *non*drug-induced mystical experience) were evaluated:

1. Unity

2. Transcendence of space and time

3. Deeply felt positive mood

4. A sense of sacredness

5. Objectivity and reality (*real* and *known*)

6. Paradoxicality (*empty* and *full*, *alive* and *dead*, *microscopic* and *macroscopic*)—"both / and"

7. Alleged ineffability (the realization that words can't describe the experience)

8. Transiency (the experience is temporary)

9. Persisting positive changes in attitude and behavior

50. Was the Marsh Chapel experiment successful?

The results of our experiment would indicate that psilocybin is an important tool for the study of the mystical state of consciousness. Our data would suggest that such an overwhelming experience . . . can possibly be therapeutic if approached and worked with in a sensitive and adequate way.

—Walter Pahnke, *"Drugs and Mysticism," International Journal of Parapsychology, at http://www.erowid.org/entheogens/journals/ entheogens_journal3.shtml*

Results were very positively in favor of psilocybin inducing a mystical or spiritual experience. Nine out of ten of the students who received the psilocybin had a full-fledged spiritual experience, compared to just one of the placebo group. Furthermore, in a follow-up to the experiment, conducted 25 years later, the students who had been given the psilocybin all recalled the experience as having been one of the high points of their spiritual lives and confirmed the "trip" as having elements of a mystical nature.

51. When did Timothy Leary first experiment with LSD?

An interview with Reverend Randall Laakko, one of the 10 participants in the study who received psilocybin rather than the placebo, can be seen at

ON THE WEB

http://www.youtube.com/watch?v= DxDZW6n69-0

A movie trailer titled *Walter Pahnke and the Good Friday Experiment* is available at

http://www.youtube.com/watch?v= G6mlyt34-gc

Pahnke's first-hand account of the Marsh Chapel experiment, including procedural details, data tables, and documentation can be read at

PRACTICAL TIP

http://www.erowid.org/entheogens/jour- nals/entheogens_journal3.shtml

Timothy Leary experienced his first LSD "trip" in 1962, courtesy of British researcher Michael Hollingshead, who was among Leary's associates and colleagues at Harvard. Leary declared the trip to be "the most shattering experience of my life"; he and Alpert expanded their research to encompass LSD experiments and founded an organization called the International Federation for Internal Freedom (IFIF). Together with the flamboyant Hollingshead, who is credited with introducing many celebrities to acid, they began to distribute the drugs to a wider variety of people, including writers, musicians, and artists—all well-known names from the Beat

Generation: Allen Ginsberg, Arthur Koestler, Jack Kerouac, Abbie Hoffman, William S. Burroughs, Neal Cassady, Thelonius Monk, Charles Mingus, Marshall McLuhan, among others, who used insights garnered from their experiences to shape their creative talents.

52. Why did Leary leave Harvard?

Leary and Alpert were both fired from their respective lecturer/professor positions on the faculty at Harvard in the spring of 1963. The University's official statement cited "failure to keep classroom appointments and absenteeism from Cambridge without permission" on the part of Leary and dismissed Alpert for allegedly giving psilocybin mushrooms to undergraduate students who were not enrolled in the formal study; however, these are more than likely "convenient charges" leveled against the perpetrators of an increasingly embarrassing and uncomfortable position for the school with regard to the public attention and controversy surrounding LSD.

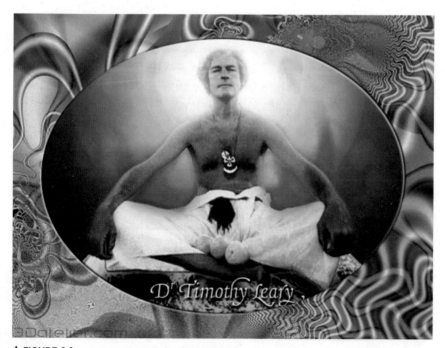

▲ FIGURE 6.3

Dr. Timothy Leary, often called the High Priest of the psychedelic movement.
SOURCE: http://uncyclopedia.wikia.com/wiki/File:Psych-Tim-Leary.jpg#file. wiki commons license.

Timothy Leary's Trip Thru Time is an image-rich slideshow; each slide opens to a video of an interview with Leary, a public appearance or lecture by Leary, or a documentary about Leary; there are also READ MORE links that display text of writings and quotes by and about Leary:

http://timothyleary.org/#1

Leary and Alpert continued their research privately at Leary's home, Millbrook Estate, where they were frequently joined by Hollingshead, Ginsberg, and others. Beat poet Allen Ginsberg supported the belief of the researchers that psychedelic substances could help people achieve a higher level of consciousness, which they termed "turning on," and, together with Leary, began to encourage other intellectuals and artists to try the psychedelics.

> *"Turn on" meant go within to activate your neural and genetic equipment. Become sensitive to the many and various levels of consciousness and the specific triggers that engage them. Drugs were one way to accomplish this end. "Tune in" meant interact harmoniously with the world around you—externalize, materialize, express your new internal perspectives. "Drop out" suggested an active, selective, graceful process of detachment from involuntary or unconscious commitments. "Drop Out" meant self-reliance, a discovery of one's singularity, a commitment to mobility, choice, and change. Unhappily, my explanations of this sequence of personal development were often misinterpreted to mean "Get stoned and abandon all constructive activity."*
>
> *—Timothy Leary, Flashbacks: A Personal and Cultural History of an Era, at http://en.wikipedia.org/wiki/Turn_on,_tune_in,_drop_out*

The use of psychedelics, on escaping the confines of the research clinics, gathered momentum like a snowball rolling downhill. By the mid-to-late 1960s, recreational use by students as well as the "invited visionaries" had sunk a toehold; the psychedelic movement was well under way.

Our next chapter will discuss the events and issues that confronted the psychedelic movement once it became "too popular."

Promising Research Grinds to a Halt

Yes, the psychedelic movement was well under way, but it was a short-lived voyage. Now, some 50 years later, it seems almost as though it was just a fad, especially considering the multitude of significant and remarkable advancements that have been made in the field of medical research in that time. It is important to remember that the advent of LSD was actually responsible for many advances in neuroscience; LSD research provided a major source of information for the discovery of the serotonin neurotransmitter system.

In this chapter we will discuss why research into psychedelics as a tool for psychotherapy was discontinued, and we will make some comparisons between psychedelics and presently recognized psychotherapeutic drugs. We will also learn about clinical studies and certain strictures of the US Food and Drug Administration (FDA) and the US Drug Enforcement Administration (DEA).

> **NOTE**
>
> In 1954, the structural relationship between LSD and serotonin was recognized by Woolley and Shaw, chemists from the Rockefeller Institute for Medical Research, and the mental effects of LSD were studied for interactions with serotonin in the brain. These studies appear to be "the first formal recognition that perhaps brain chemistry had something to do with behavior, and particularly with mental illness. That was what one might call an 'ah-ha moment!' Suddenly, the role of brain chemistry became of more than academic interest."—David E. Nichols, PhD, "Serotonin, and the Past and Future of LSD"; *www.maps.org/news-letters/v23n1/ v23n1_p20-23.pdf*

53. Why did promising research stop?

The simple answer to that question is that research slowed down because the drugs became classified as illegal in the United States in the mid-1960s and were, therefore, banned. The scientific community no longer had legal or easy access to these compounds. Neuroscientists, researchers, and the psychiatric and pharmaceutical communities focused their attention on other methods of therapy and the development of legal psychoactive drugs.

The reasons the drugs achieved illegal status are more numerous and more complicated; several factors combined to contribute to the situation: the times, the US government, and ironically, the very people who were the psychedelics' loudest and most avid proponents were among those who unintentionally brought research efforts to a halt.

54. What was it about the times that contributed to the ban on these drugs?

The 1960s and early '70s were a turbulent period in American history, and the psychedelic "scene" was very much a part of that turbulence, playing against the Cuban Missile Crisis and the threat of nuclear war; the assassination of President John F. Kennedy; the Vietnam "conflict" and the growing, resounding antiwar sentiment; the civil rights movement and, later in the decade, the assassination of Martin Luther King; the feminist movement; the Kent State massacre; the speculation surrounding covert CIA activities (spooks among us!); the assassination of Robert Kennedy; the Space Race. It was a time of social contention and unrest, a tinderbox atmosphere aflame with every kind of protest and demonstration—sit-ins, strikes, marches, flag burnings. Young voters felt distrust and disillusionment in a government that drafted young men and sent them to be killed or maimed in a questionable, arguable war and in a legislature that was tediously slow in equalizing rights for women and blacks and other minorities. "Conspiracy theories" surrounding the assassination of JFK further increased disillusionment and distrust. The antiestablishment, nonmaterialistic philosophies of the "Beat Generation" intellectuals, writers, and poets of the mid-to-late-1950s inspired a cultural phenomenon that flared on college campuses in the early '60s and was further fueled by the entheogenic properties of the psychedelics, which were being disseminated freely. Leary's advice to "Question Authority" seemed appropriate, and "Make Love, Not War" made so much more sense than nuclear war. The well-educated Beat writers paved the way for the hippies and the flower children, whose recreational use of consciousness-raising drugs proliferated too quickly, without the restraints and controls that were present in clinical use.

For more information about the Beat Generation and the intellectuals and writers who inspired the cultural consciousness of the 1960s, there's a brief, well-written article at *http://www.online-literature. com/periods/beat.php*

PRACTICAL TIP

55. What was the US government's role?

We've discussed that the US government was the target of the consciousness-aware demonstrators of the antiwar, civil rights, and women's movements. By instituting the CIA's MK-Ultra Program (mentioned in Chapter 6, "Psychedelic Research and Pioneers in the mid-1900s"), which used the mind-altering compounds for studies in mind control, the government also played a direct role in what resulted in the ban on psychedelics. The MK-Ultra project included many substudies, and although not all involved the use of drugs, it was a large project that infiltrated several dozens of institutions—

In the 1950s and early 1960s, the agency gave mind-altering drugs to hundreds of unsuspecting Americans in an effort to explore the possibilities of controlling human consciousness. Many of the human guinea pigs were mental patients, prisoners, drug addicts, and prostitutes—"people who could not fight back," as one agency officer put it. In one case, a mental patient in Kentucky was dosed with LSD continuously for 174 days. . . . First-hand testimony, fragmentary government documents, and court records show that at least one participant died, others went mad, and still others suffered psychological damage after participating in the project . . . (Tim Weiner, *The New York Times,* March 10, 1999).

including more than forty colleges and universities, as well as hospitals, prisons, and pharmaceutical companies. Understandably, a project of such size required employing several hundred people; it is not surprising that psychedelic compounds—particularly LSD—passed through countless hands affiliated with the program, were disbursed across college campuses, and made their way to the general population. So, intentionally or not, the government was responsible for the spread in the use of psychedelics both by providing the drugs themselves and by fostering a sociopolitical climate that was in need of change—change that seemed possible through the transformative qualities of the psychedelics.

Fascinating stories of psychedelic history can be found in *Acid Dreams. The Complete Social History of LSD: The CIA, the Sixties and Beyond* by Martin A. Lee and Bruce Shalin, New York: Grove Press, 1992.

There was a good deal of subterfuge and covert activity surrounding the MK-Ultra program, and several deaths. It is arguably one of the most heinous projects ever conducted by the US government, and as stories about the project trickled out, there was more cause for distrust in the "establishment."

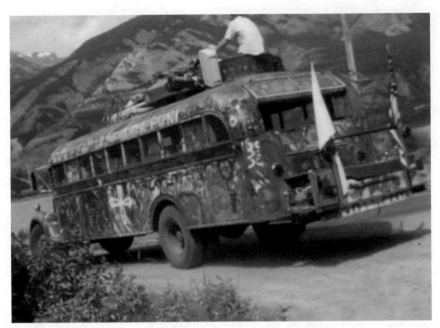

▲ **FIGURE 7.1**
"Furthur" was the name of this 1939 International Harvester bus bought by Ken Kesey and his "Merry Band of Pranksters." Painted garrishly and fully supplied with psychedelics, the Merry Pranksters drove from California to New York and back in 1964. Photo (1964) by Rcarlberg via Wikimedia Commons.

Author Ken Kesey was a subject in the MK-Ultra project while a student at Stanford, working at the Menlo Park State Psychiatric Hospital as a night porter. In his case, Kesey was aware that he was being given drugs; he was a paid volunteer. When tested with LSD, his response was to smuggle the drug home with him and have parties that he called "Acid Tests." It is said that he wrote parts of his best seller *One Flew Over the Cuckoo's Nest* while on LSD.

CIA Mind Control Operation MK ULTRA is a full-length ABC News documentary filmed in the 1970s. It offers great detail about MK-Ultra and includes interviews with some of the researchers and victims who were involved in the projects: *http://www.youtube.com/watch?v=2t-L26MjwRo*

Shorter videos include *The Five Most Shocking CIA Experiments of Project MKUltra*, which can be seen at *http://www.youtube.com/watch?v=7ff24-xGrSI* and, also titled *CIA Mind Control Operation MK ULTRA*, at *http://www.youtube.com/watch?v=i46RI2twVao*

ON THE WEB

56. What did proponents of the psychedelic movement do to interfere with research?

In the late 1950s and early 1960s, Sandoz laboratories, where LSD-25 was created, wanted to increase the interest of the psychiatric community in the product and were happy to make it available free of charge to those who wanted to use it; this of course spurred worldwide distribution. And the Johnny Appleseed of LSD, Al Hubbard, whom we met in Chapter 6, enthusiastically carried his leather satchel from Sandoz Laboratories in Basel, Switzerland, far and wide. So, the drug wasn't difficult to obtain. Convinced that if everyone could experience, as Huxley put it, "Love as the primary and fundamental cosmic fact," it would bring peace to the world, Timothy Leary and writers Ken Kesey, Allen Ginsberg, Jack Kerouac, William S. Burroughs, and others of the Beat genre who had felt spiritual expansiveness from the entheogenic effects of the psychedelics were enthusiastically bent on sharing the experience widely; the psychedelics escaped the confines of clinics and laboratories and began to be distributed widely. Once LSD, psilocybin, and peyote found their way onto college campuses as recreational drugs, the scientific community lost control of the use of the substances that, for the previous couple of decades, had been theirs. These were no longer compounds solely for research, they had become a quick fix for soul searchers, and their transcendental properties transcended the research laboratories and clinics.

57. What was the problem with the psychedelics being used recreationally?

It is estimated that, by 1964, over four million people in the United States had used LSD outside of proper medical treatment centers, and negative publicity and grossly exaggerated horror stories about the drug and its properties began to appear. By 1966, tens of millions of people worldwide had used the drug recreationally, and the "bad rep" of the psychedelics grew. Many academic and spiritual leaders at the time proposed a system of control that would allow for the safe use of the drug, however, the authorities made LSD illegal. As with other drugs, this legislation did little to curb LSD's recreational use, but the move effectively halted practically all of medical research on the drug. Doctors and scientists, unlike the hippies who had no qualms about taking a banned drug, could not associate their professional work with illegal substances, and as medical licenses to use LSD experimentally became more difficult to acquire, many interested physicians and researchers moved on to other projects—such as the new antipsychotics that the growing pharmaceutical industry was beginning to push aggressively.

These were—and are—potent drugs; taken indiscriminately and unguided—without regard for dosage, set and setting, they could be dangerous; they *can* be dangerous. It is not the intent of the authors to suggest that a new generation should pick up where the hippies left off in terms of the consumption of psychedelics. To the contrary, it was the wide-spread and inappropriate use of LSD, magic mushrooms, and peyote that hampered what could have been decades of significant progress in the field of psychiatry and in the neurosciences. Keeping in mind that the study of LSD contributed significantly to the understanding of the neurotransmitter system, who can even imagine what might have been discovered about the human brain in this length of time? Research and development of the psychedelics are almost a half century behind the development of other pharmaceuticals such as antidepressants, mood stabilizers, and antipsychotics; this is paradoxical, considering the fact that the naturally occurring psychoactives have been around for thousands of years, whereas the exogenous chemicals now being manufactured into psychopharmaceuticals are so very, very new.

58. What exactly are controlled substances?

The term **controlled substance** means a drug or other substance, or immediate precursor, included in schedule I, II, III, IV, or V . . . The term does not include distilled spirits, wine, malt beverages, or tobacco; those terms are defined or used in subtitle E of the Internal Revenue Code of 1986.—*http://www.fda.gov/ regulatoryinformation/legislation/ucm148726 .htm#cntlsbb*

DEFINITION

President Richard Nixon signed into law the Comprehensive Drug Abuse Prevention and Control Act of 1970, which includes as Title II the **Controlled Substances Act (CSA)**. According to the US Department of Justice Drug Enforcement Administration, Office of Diversion Control, drugs and other substances that are considered controlled substances under the CSA are divided into five schedules. Both the **Drug Enforcement Administration (DEA)** and the **Food and Drug Administration (FDA)**, determine which substances are added to or removed from the various schedules. Substances are placed in their respective schedules (Schedule I being the most harmful, Schedule V being the least harmful) based on whether they have a currently accepted medical use in treatment in the United States, their relative potential to be abused, and the likelihood of their causing dependence (addiction) when abused.

"Please note that a substance need not be listed as a controlled substance to be treated as a Schedule I substance for criminal prosecution."—*http://www.justice.gov/dea/druginfo/ds.shtml*

We list the description of Schedule I because it includes the psychedelics, which are our focus. Descriptions of each schedule level and lists of all the controlled substances can be found at *http://www.deadiversion.usdoj.gov/schedules/#list* or at *http://www.fda.gov/regulatoryinformation/legislation/ucm148726.htm* (this FDA site provides the complete text of the Controlled Substances Act, and the schedules are more thoroughly complete).

You will find certain drugs such as cocaine, methamphetamine, and others that are far more addictive than psychedelics listed on lower-level schedules.

According to the DEA,

Schedule I drugs, substances, or chemicals are defined as drugs with no currently accepted medical use and a high potential for abuse. Schedule I drugs are the most dangerous drugs of all the drug schedules, with potentially severe psychological or physical dependence.

Schedule I drugs include

- Heroin
- lysergic acid diethylamide (LSD)
- marijuana (cannabis)
- 3,4-methylenedioxymethamphetamine (ecstasy)
- Methaqualone
- peyote

59. How do psychedelics compare with other controlled substances?

The decision by the authorities to list LSD, cannabis, and peyote as Schedule I substances would appear to be an overreaction to the recreational abuse of the drugs in the '60s and a typical bureaucratic response to the Nixon administration's launch of the **War on Drugs** (1971) rather than a classification based on factual representation of the drugs' properties. First, that these drugs have "no currently accepted medical use" could be in large part because they are illegal; researchers and doctors have been reluctant or unable to acquire them; research has inched forward, but progress is not what it could be if there were more cooperation from the government authorities. Second, the potential for "severe psychological or physical dependence" is actually quite low with psychedelics: physiological impairment is slight; mild fluctuations in pulse and blood pressure and dilation of the pupils are almost all that can be expected with LSD. With MDMA (ecstasy) and cannabis, bodily relaxation is probably the most notable physical experience. These compounds are not physically addictive; however, the transcendant feelings of peaceful uplifting might be powerful enough to encourage repeated use, especially with cannabis. A drug with more powerful physical effects and higher addictive qualities is alcohol, which—together with nicotine—is not a *controlled* substance and is therefore not on any of the schedules. Nicotine, as is well known, is quite addictive and can cause irreparable physiological damage.

"FDA Consumer Advice on Powdered Pure Caffeine"

NOTE

The FDA is warning about powdered pure caffeine being marketed directly to consumers, and recommends avoiding these products. In particular, the FDA is concerned about powdered pure caffeine sold in bulk bags over the Internet.

These products are essentially 100 percent caffeine. A single teaspoon of pure caffeine is roughly equivalent to the amount in 25 cups of coffee.

Pure caffeine is a powerful stimulant and very small amounts may cause accidental overdose. Parents should be aware that these products may be attractive to young people.

Pure caffeine products are potentially dangerous, and serious adverse events can result, including death. People with preexisting heart conditions should not use them.—*www.fda.gov/Food/RecallsOutbreaksEmergencies/SafetyAlertsAdvisories/ucm405787.htm*

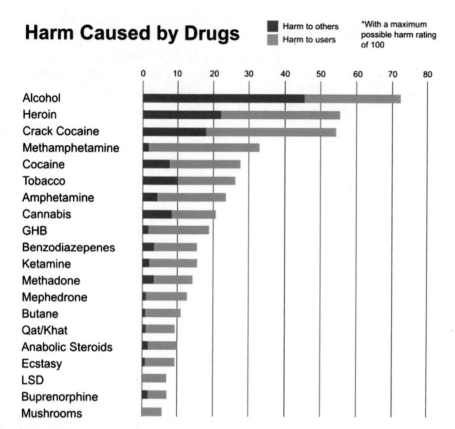

Harm Caused by Drugs

■ Harm to others
■ Harm to users

*With a maximum possible harm rating of 100

A FIGURE 7.2

Comparison of the perceived harm for various psychoactive drugs from a poll among medical psychiatrists who specialize in addiction treatment.
SOURCE: Prof. David Nutt, FMedSci, Leslie King, PhD, William Saulsbury, MA, and Colin Blakemore, FRS. "Development of a Rational Scale to Assess the Harm of Drugs of Potential Misuse." *The Lancet* 2007, 369:1047–1053. Full article available at doi:10.1016/S0140-6736(07)60464-4. wiki commons license.

The chart in Figure 7.2, developed by a group of experts in the United Kingdom, shows the relative dependence and harm among several chemical—though not necessarily controlled—substances; note the placement of tobacco and alcohol.

As do the United States and other countries, the UK assesses pharmaceuticals on the basis of harm, and some assessments might seem arbitrary. For the development of this nine-category,

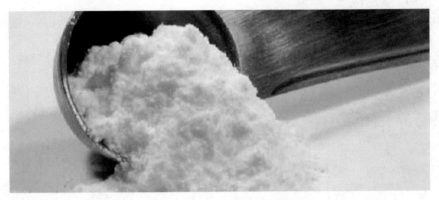

▲ FIGURE 7.3
Pure caffeine products are potentially dangerous and can result in death. This much powdered pure caffeine is the same as drinking 25 cups of coffee.
SOURCE: Image courtesy of the US Food and Drug Administration.

harm-based ranking for recreational drugs, the authors of the matrix collaborated with psychiatrists registered as specialists in addiction in the UK's Royal College of Psychiatrists register; with experts whose experiences were in other specialized areas of addiction, including chemistry, pharmacology, and forensic science; and with legal and police services. As with the US CSA schedule rankings, some drugs' placements under the UK's Misuse of Drugs Act do not coincide with the opinions of experts in the field of physical and mental addiction.

Note also that caffeine does not appear at all on the chart. Yet, the homepage of the FDA website features a photo and a warning: "Pure caffeine products are potentially dangerous and can result in death." Of course, the warning is with regard to powdered *pure* caffeine; however, coffee fanatics, tea fanciers, and cola guzzlers had best be aware that yes, caffeine *is* a drug.

60. How does a drug become approved and legal?

Many clinical treatments in medicine first arise out of accidental anecdotal experience. Many others arise because a pharmaceutical company has specifically designed a new chemical with a particular target in mind. When a new chemical emerges in this way, there must be preclinical studies to test whether the chemical is safe to give to humans. Once adequate testing for preclinical studies has been completed, the process continues to clinical studies. These and other details with regard to research will be discussed in the following chapters.

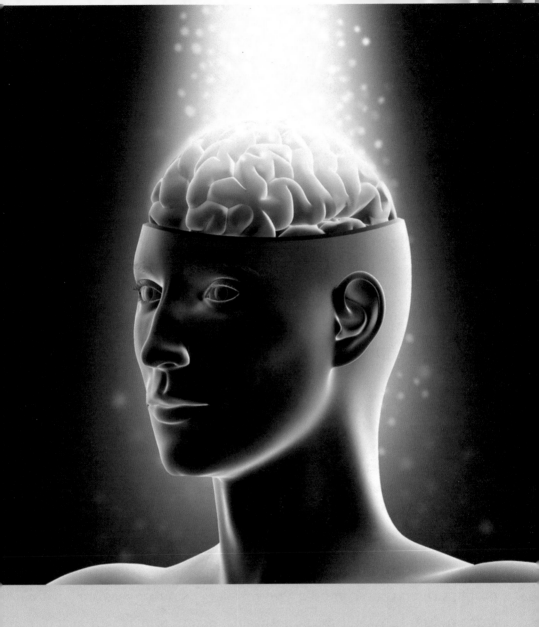

PART THREE

Current Research

In these chapters we take a look at research that is ongoing at this time and the standards and procedures mandated by the governing regulatory bodies. Chapter 8 outlines the clinical trial process that is necessary before a drug can be brought to market. Chapter 9 discusses "Current Research," the illnesses being studied and the psychedelic drugs that are being tested to assist with therapy for these conditions. Chapter 10 attempts to cover information about medical marijuana studies that are being developed and explains why medical marijuana research is so slow to gain acceptance.

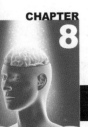

CHAPTER 8

Making Pharmaceuticals Legally Available

61. How does a drug become an FDA-approved, legal medicine?

As mentioned at the end of Chapter 7, many clinical treatments in medicine stem from accidental experiences or because a pharmaceutical company has designed a new chemical to treat a specific condition or disease. When a new chemical appears likely to become beneficial to the medical community, there are **preclinical studies** that must be carried out in order to test whether the chemical is safe to be given to humans. These include **in vitro** (studies that are performed on cells or biological molecules outside their normal biological context) tests, which involve adding concentrations of the chemical to isolated slices of tissues (heart, lungs, kidneys, brain, etc.) to determine the drug's toxicity. The new chemical will also be tested against animal models in order to provide further information about safety and toxicity. Once preclinical studies have proven successful and it is determined that the new drug can be safely administered to humans, the **clinical studies** (also called **clinical trials**) begin.

62. What is involved in a clinical study?

Clinical trials for the development of new drugs normally encompass four phases over the course of many years. The drug must be tested for safety, effectiveness, side effects, tolerability, interaction with other chemical compounds and/or foods, possibility of allergic reaction, appropriate administration (i.e., dosage, time of day, with or without eating food, age appropriateness, etc.). If the drug successfully passes through Phases I, II, and III, it will usually be approved by the FDA for use among the general population.

63. What are the four phases?

The first, or **Phase I clinical studies**, involve testing the drug on *healthy* human volunteers; that is, people who do not have the specific disorder the drug is intended to treat. The purpose of such tests is to gather information about appropriate safe doses and effects of the new drug. Volunteers, often students at a university where the research is being carried out, are usually paid for their services. (Recall Ken Kesey's volunteering for the CIA's MK-Ultra program while a student at Stanford.)

Phase II studies involve small-scale clinical trials in which the drug is given to small groups of patients who do have the disorder being tested. Between 10 to 40 people is usual, though sometimes groups as large as 100 people participate. Many Phase II studies follow the protocol for a **double-blind, placebo-controlled, randomized study.** Phase II studies use the data collected from the Phase I studies with regard to safe dosage and other information in order to develop a standard, best-practices procedure for administering the drug.

After phase two come **Phase III clinical trials**, in which the established, best-treatment protocol for the new drug is rolled out to larger groups for wide-scale testing on clinical patients. In this way, many hundreds of patients receive treatment under a standardized protocol to ensure uniform results.

After successfully completing Phase III trials, **Phase IV** puts the drug on the market under a very restricted license. Thousands of patients will be able to use it in an open-label fashion (that is, they know what they are taking, rather than taking it blindly), and their doctors will closely monitor the process. Effects—particularly any adverse effects—are documented by the physicians and reported to the drug company.

64. What is the double-blind, placebo-controlled, randomized study?

Clinical studies must be rigorously designed to reduce as many aspects of bias as possible. The gold standard for drug development is the double-blind, placebo-controlled, randomized study. Recall from Chapter 6 that the Marsh Chapel experiment was one of the most thoroughly designed double-blind, placebo-controlled studies of its day. In this type of study, identically matched subjects are randomly assigned to a control group or to an experimental group. The people in the control group receive the placebo (a dummy; an inert compound) and the experimental group gets the active drug (the drugs look identical).

It can take between five and twenty years to bring a drug to market in this way. Today, the average cost of getting a brand new drug to market is around $125 million US dollars.

NOTE

The study is called "double-blind" because neither the subjects nor the examiners who will be doing the testing know which group is the control group (taking the placebo) or the experimental group (taking the active drug). In this way, differences seen in outcomes between the two groups can be put down entirely to the physiological action of the drug and cannot be attributed to other influences.

65. What is meant by "set and setting," and why are they important?

Although nonaddictive and relatively safe physiologically, the psychological effects of LSD and other potent psychedelics can be dangerous; the misuse of these drugs can cause harm. The depth of the psychedelic experience can be frightening and disorientating for the user. For many ill-prepared users, the experience can provoke anxiety and overwhelming feelings of panic and loss of control—what have been termed as **bad trips**. The importance of **set and setting** and guidance through experiences, as well as dosage, cannot be overstated.

A lesson learned very early in the 1950s is that the totality of the experience encompasses more factors than merely the choice of psychedelic drug used or the dosage taken. The concepts of set and setting are essential. Set refers to the user's mindset, and setting refers to the environment in which the drug is taken.

Mindset includes a whole range of attitudes, beliefs, and expectations: the user's expectations about what will happen, his or her experience of the particular drug, stories and opinions of others, what the media says, awareness of the drug's physiological effects, fears and fantasies about what might happen, religious orientation, what is to be gained by taking the drug, any past experience with drugs, whether previous mental states have included nonordinary states of consciousness or issues surrounding the user's own mental health.

Setting includes the physical environment where the drug is taken, the individuals the user is with at the time, what music is played (if any), familiarity with the place, ambient temperature, comfort, physical activity at the time, whether there is a suitable length of time to enjoy the experience before having to "get back to real life," and even broader issues such as what the social climate and attitude toward drugs is in the environment—how many other people will be around, is it party time or an intimate gathering or a therapy session, is there an atmosphere of expectation, a sense of judgment?

Set and setting have such a vast effect on the overall outcome of the psychedelic experience that they absolutely cannot be disregarded. When one hears horror stories of "trips" that have gone wrong, it is invariably because lack of attention was paid to these factors.

Case Study

The following story of what might be considered a "bad trip" on psilocybin was told to one of the authors by an acquaintance. It is an example of misuse; the user was, unfortunately, not guided by someone knowledgeable, was not prepared with forewarning of the "at one with the universe" experience particular to psychedelics, and was not familiar with dosage. Set and setting are dubious; natural surroundings can be conducive to a rewarding experience if the user is adequately prepared otherwise.

On a Sunday afternoon in the spring, a friend and I drove out to the wildlife refuge on an island close to where we lived. Here, a seven-mile length of narrow dirt road stretching across salt pannes, marsh, sand dunes, hillocks, and meadows ran parallel to the coastline and a pristine beach. It was a drive we loved, and we thought it would be so cool to eat these magic 'shrooms my friend had gotten and enjoy being surrounded by peace and quiet and nature full blown. One of our favorite walks was through Hellcat Swamp. The Parks Service had built a boardwalk that rambled out over the marsh, and we often saw waterfowl—egrets, ducks, geese, herons—and the occasional land animal—deer, fox—venturing out from the scrubby brush on the east side of the swamp. We ate the mushrooms at home because we did not live far, and sure enough, just as we parked near the entrance to Hellcat, I began to feel a sort of "wavy" feeling. The sky became kind of opalescent, and leaves on the bushes that lined the path leading to the boardwalk shimmered, sort of. "Way cool," I thought. As we started along the boardwalk, I felt curiously light and my feet seemed not to touch the boardwalk. We came upon a beaver dam and stared at it for what seemed like hours, and it seemed that I could see into it—like I could see the beavers working and paddling with their tails. Cat-o'-nine tails chimed lowly as they bowed gracefully in the breeze, sounding at once like high, tinkling wind chimes and the deep bellow of low-pitched organ pipes.

We hadn't ever taken magic mushrooms before. We really had little knowledge of them except that they might cause altered perceptions of things. We didn't know how many to eat.

Everything shimmered and shined. It was so lovely to be a part of the marsh, a part of the sky and the beavers and the cattails. Colors became so vivid that I felt I was tucked in a box of Crayola 64. The ocean on the other side of the road heaved and roared and the waves rushed in and out of my ears and suddenly I wasn't me anymore, I had dissolved into the beauty and wildness of Hellcat Swamp—and I couldn't handle it. Where had "I" gone?

"Please, we have to go" . . . I whispered to my friend. "I feel like my soul is leaving my body . . . Please let's get home . . ." I began to panic; I'd never had an experience like that before. I was so far out of my element . . . I kept thinking of a poem I remembered—over and over I thought, "the world is too much with

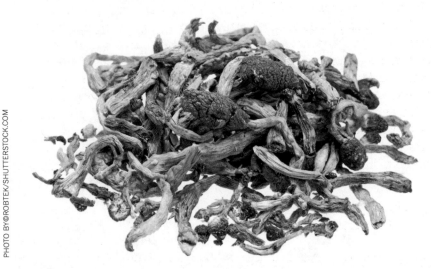

▲ **FIGURE 8.1**
Dried psilocybin mushrooms.

us . . ." too much, too much . . . I couldn't relax. I knew it would pass soon enough, but I couldn't enjoy it. I didn't feel grounded or centered. Everything I saw was so lovely . . . silky leaves and tree trunks of velvet and iridescence touching everything, but I had not known I would lose myself in it . . .

I wished we were with someone who had some experience with what I was feeling—someone who could help me sort out this inexplicable lightness and the knowing that green isn't green but is all colors, sparkling, and feeling part of it all. I did not feel safe and I wanted to go home where nature wouldn't grab at me like that. I wanted to lie down on a couch and let my mind just wander. I did not want to be walking on—or floating above—a boardwalk with so many distractions around me—birds, trees, sunshine, ocean waves, cattails. It was all too much. Too much.

66. Do psychedelics go through the same clinical-trial process that other pharmaceuticals go through?

Yes, they do. The FDA standards are strict, which is to the benefit of patients and general consumers. Although it's a lengthy process, each step is necessary in order to avoid bringing harmful medicines to pharmacy shelves. The health and well-being of all of us do not allow shortcuts.

However, in the case of psychedelics, consider the fact that LSD, MDMA, and others are chemicals that have been used by humans for dozens of years—and cannabis and peyote, thousands of years. So there is more than enough reliable evidence to maintain that these substances are not toxic for humans, but it is largely anecdotal evidence.

Furthermore, because they are controlled or illegal drugs, it is all the more difficult to obtain government sanction to work with them. The strict regulatory processes for this kind of research and the government's withholding of approval makes bringing these drugs to market prohibitively costly and takes many years; ironically, these compounds, known to be nontoxic and physiologically harmless, might take longer to reach the psychiatric community's clinics than newly designed antipsychotics and antidepressants—the majority of which are accompanied by long lists of warnings of possible dangerous side effects—that are touted by the pharmaceutical companies.

67. Are any psychedelics currently undergoing clinical studies?

Yes. Although LSD was made illegal in 1966, *research* itself was *not* banned. Its criminalized status made LSD extremely difficult to obtain, however, so the amount of research dwindled to a near halt, and only a handful of researchers and psychotherapists continued to work with reserves of the drug that they had on hand.

MDMA is not one of the classic psychedelics, but it was fated to follow the same path as LSD. In 1976, a new method of synthesizing MDMA, which was *not* scheduled as an illegal substance at that time, was developed by chemist Alexander Shulgin (see Chapter 1), who introduced the drug to Leo Zeff, a retired psychedelic psychotherapist who had been forced by circumstances to discontinue his work with LSD. Zeff promoted the drug to fellow members of the psychiatric community, and MDMA began to be used both therapeutically and recreationally in the late 1970s, gaining in popularity on into the early 1980s. A new, legal alternative to LSD for psychedelic therapy had been discovered. As its recreational use proliferated among the **rave culture**, however, the US DEA began to collect information about abuses of ecstasy; the ban was imposed in 1985.

The ban on MDMA was strongly protested by a group of psychotherapists who had been using the empathogen effectively in their practices. This group pressured the courts and the DEA for the ability to continue research, convinced that the drug had important medical uses and should not be on the controlled substances Schedule I. From this group emerged the Multidisciplinary Association for Psychedelic Studies (MAPS), founded by Rick Doblin, PhD, in 1986. Since its inception, MAPS has campaigned tirelessly for evidence-based research to justify clinical use of MDMA and other psychedelic drugs and cannabis, and though there have been—and continue to be—difficult battles, several studies are now under way.

Through the auspices of MAPS, a study on LSD has been completed, as announced in the *New York Times* in March 2014.

The study was the first double-blind, placebo-controlled study of the therapeutic use of LSD in human beings since the early

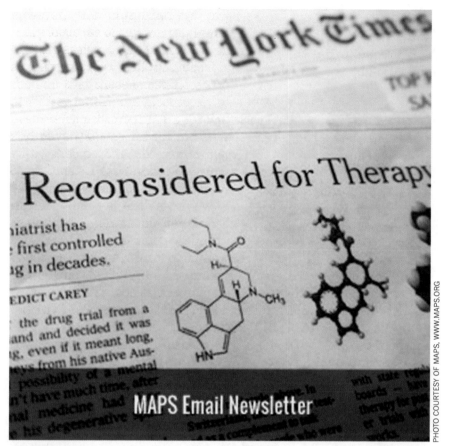

▲ FIGURE 8.2
March 3, 2014. This morning, the *New York Times* announced today's publication of the first study of the therapeutic use of LSD in humans in over 40 years. (*http://www. nytimes.com/2014/03/04/health/lsd-reconsidered-for-therapy.html?_r=0*). Published online (*http://www.maps.org/research-archive/lsd/Gasser-2014-JMND-4March14.pdf*) in the *Journal of Nervous and Mental Disease*, the study is a historic turning point for psychedelic science and medicine, marking the end of four decades of research taboo. SOURCE: Email from Brad Burge, MAPS Director of Communications and Marketing.

1970s. The Phase II trials investigated the safety and efficacy of LSD-assisted psychotherapy for anxiety associated with life-threatening diseases.

68. Is the MAPS organization just a group of former "hippies"?

It is important to stress that MAPS is an international, professional organization for the scientific, educational, medical, and psychiatric communities; the group does not lobby for legal use of the compounds for recreation. MAPS is alive and flourishing and still led by Rick Doblin. Without the voice of MAPS, there is little doubt that the pursuit of psychedelics for therapy might have died by the end of the 1980s. Following, the MAPS mission statement:

MAPS is a [nonprofit] research and educational organization that develops medical, legal, and cultural contexts for people to benefit from the careful uses of psychedelics and marijuana. MAPS furthers its mission by:

- Developing psychedelics and marijuana into prescription medicines.
- Training therapists and working to establish a network of treatment centers.
- Supporting scientific research into spirituality, creativity, and neuroscience.
- Educating the public honestly about the risks and benefits of psychedelics and marijuana.

MAPS envisions a world where psychedelics and marijuana are safely and legally available for beneficial uses, and where research is governed by rigorous scientific evaluation of their risks and benefits.

MAPS values encompass

- *Transparency*—Information is shared openly and clearly. Communications are respectful, honest, and forthright.
- *Passion and Perseverance*—We persist in the face of challenges. We have a sense of urgency about our work, and know that it's a long-term effort.
- *Intelligent Risk*—Our decisions are informed by research. We try new things and learn from our mistakes.
- *Trust and Accountability*—We value integrity and honesty, and embrace high standards.

— *http://www.maps.org/about/mission*

69. Is all current research supported by MAPS?

Because of limited resources, MAPS can support only a small number of studies. MAPS-sponsored research has included, and still does include, studies on LSD, ibogaine, psilocybin, and ayahuasca;

however, the organization's primary focus (as of this writing) is on MDMA-assisted psychotherapy as a treatment for PTSD, because it is thought that these substances and this disorder are the most likely to eventually achieve FDA approval and pave the way for future work with other psychedelics and other conditions. Posttraumatic stress is a major worldwide concern, particularly (but not exclusively) with regard to veterans of the armed services. There is much publicity about the serious nature of chronic

 For information about research efforts and educational resources, many of which are available free, online, please visit MAPS at

www.maps.org

 "We hope that once the FDA approves MDMA for use as an adjunct to psychotherapy for PTSD, the door will open for research into psychedelics as treatments for other conditions as well as into their neuroscientific, spiritual, and creative uses."—MAPS FAQs; www.maps.org

PTSD, and its sufferers are often so disabled by the disorder that traditional methods of therapy are slow or ineffective; suicide frequently becomes the last resort for these patients. MDMA is a logical choice as a "favorite" psychedelic for the MAPS focus (for many reasons, which we will discuss in the following chapter) because several studies of MDMA by researchers in many countries were under way at the time MDMA was banned and MAPS was founded. The wealth of these research data allows research to continue without the need to repeat early studies for safety and toxicity.

70. What are some other organizations that are studying psychedelics?

There are studies being conducted that are not affiliated with MAPS. Most of these are in the Phase I clinical trials, in which psychedelics are administered to healthy subjects in order to learn more about the effects of these drugs. Research has been and is still conducted at several hospitals, universities, and institutes in the United States and in Europe, New Zealand, Mexico, and much research is sponsored by foundations such as the Albert Hofmann Foundation, the Heffter Research Institute, the Beckley Foundation, and the Promind Foundation, and some governmental bodies such as the European Commission, the Netherlands Organization for Scientific Research, Swiss National Science Foundation, National Institute on Drug Abuse (NIDA), and the National Institute of Health (NIH). Psychedelics being studied in addition to MDMA include LSD, DMT, ibogaine, ayahuasca, *Salvia divinorum*, psilocybin, peyote, and others. We will explore recent and current research in more detail in the following chapters.

71. Are pharmaceutical companies researching psychedelics or sponsoring such research?

The unfortunate truth is that "money makes the world go around"; financial funding is necessary for all medical research, even that by the most altruistic of researchers. The protocols and the ultimate goal of psychedelic-assisted therapy are not really in the best profit-bearing interests of the multi-million-dollar pharmaceutical corporations. The goal of psychedelic-assisted therapy is to *heal* patients of their traumatic disorders through therapy enhanced by opening channels of trust and communication. The goal of pharmaceutical companies is to continue to produce and sell antidepressants and antipsychotics that will *control* a patient's disorder by masking symptoms. Contemporary medications are usually taken every day, and though they might effectively offer a significant degree of relief and help a sufferer's day-to-day functioning, they are often prescribed for months, years, or for a lifetime. In some cases, dosage is periodically increased or additional medications are added to a patient's regimen. Such a protocol of continuous medication is, obviously, more advantageous for a pharmaceutical company's bottom line than the three or four doses of a psychedelic, administered to open communication between patient and therapist, would be.

Visit *PubMed* for recent psychedelic research publications, or search *ClinicalTrials.gov*. A database archive called the *World Wide Web Psychedelic Bibliography* that includes past preclinical and clinical studies is available at

http://www.maps.org/resources/ psychedelic-bibliography

PRACTICAL TIP

72. What is the protocol for administering psychedelics to assist therapy?

Because research is relatively new and ongoing, no one protocol has been singled out as the probable best method for using psychedelics to assist with therapy. In general, the power of these drugs lies in their empathogenic qualities. Empathy is a major, well-recognized therapeutic tool and fosters a sense of feeling close to other people and understanding others' points of view. This quality allows a stronger sense of connection and trust between therapist and patient and encourages openness on the part of the patient to delve into those past experiences and/or present situations that cause depression, anxiety, and trauma. For the most part, low and infrequent doses (perhaps 4 or 5 weeks apart) of a pure psychedelic are all that is necessary to bring about effective interaction between patient and therapist. Unlike current psychoactive medications, which require a prescription from the local pharmacy and are taken independently by the patient at home, the psychedelic is administered by the therapist in a clinical setting; this ensures the patient's safety and appropriate reaction to the drug. Patients are screened for heart, blood pressure, and other physiological issues before being given the psychedelic; during the experience the patient is resting, fluids are given, physical responses are monitored, and the therapist(s) is(are) attentive to the patient's emerging consciousness and is(are) able to offer emotional support as needed. Also, the drug is unadulterated, unlike street drugs, so there are no contaminants to cause damaging physiological responses.

73. Is the experience like tripping?

As mentioned, for assisting with therapy, the psychedelic is administered by the therapist in a clinical setting; reactions are monitored, ensuring the patient's safety. Dosage is low compared to what can be found "on the street" for recreational purposes and is highly unlikely to cause hallucinations.

The intent for the use of psychedelics is that they assist with therapy for patients who are "blocked" and who resist opening their memories to revisit the cause(s) of their stress or disorder. Psychedelics are not meant to become medicines that cure without benefit of therapy, and they are not meant to mask symptoms and make one "feel happy," as antidepressants do; they are meant to open the mind, expand consciousness, and help one become more aware of ones' own feelings, thoughts, and perceptions.

Our next chapter discusses studies currently in development or in clinical Phase I or II. Disorders that might benefit from psychedelic-assisted therapy and the particular psychedelic under study for the disorder are described.

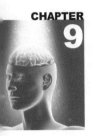

CHAPTER 9

Current Research

Keep in mind that MDMA and the classic psychedelics were originally intended for medical purposes before recreational use led to abuse; many studies were under way at the time these drugs became banned. It stands to reason that those are the studies that have continued, even if somewhat clandestinely, because there was already a considerable amount of anecdotal and preclinical data. Recall from our brief history (Chapter 6), that in the 1950s and '60s LSD was being administered to thousands of people as a treatment for alcoholism, and that the entheogenic properties of LSD, which allow spiritual growth, insight, and self-awareness, convinced Dr. Robert Sandison and others that the drug could successfully assist therapy to treat anxiety and depression. Studies in this vein have been continued, with particular interest in end-of-life anxiety and anxiety associated with life-threatening illness such as advanced-stage cancer.

Peer-reviewed papers were published in 2014 (*Journal of Psychopharmacology* and *Journal of Mental and Nervous Disease*) that describe the completed Phase II pilot study in Switzerland, which was mentioned briefly in Chapter 8. The study involved 12 subjects, 11 of whom had never taken LSD, and two LSD-assisted psychotherapy sessions; it was the first double-blind, placebo-controlled study using LSD as a therapeutic aid since the early 1970s. The study is considered successful in that significant reduction of anxiety followed the two LSD sessions and indications support the theory that LSD-assisted psychotherapy can be safely administered to humans in a clinical setting, and further research seems advisable and justified.

"MAPS' completed and future research conforms to modern drug development standards, and will help guide the development of additional research into the risks and benefits of LSD-assisted psychotherapy."—*www.maps.org*

NOTE

74. What illnesses and disorders do researchers hope to benefit from use of psychedelic-assisted therapy?

As mentioned (Chapter 8), research into one chemical compound or another frequently stems from anecdotal reports of a substance being used accidentally or after a certain amount of conjecture suggests that it might have certain properties. As we learned, research is a lengthy process. The following ailments have been or

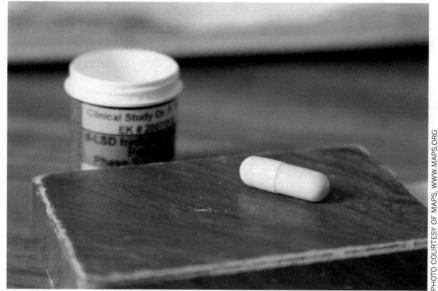

▲ FIGURE 9.1

"Experimental LSD capsule from our completed Swiss pilot study."—*www.maps.org*

are currently being researched because intentional or accidental experimentation led to further inquiry about the possible benefit of using psychedelics for their treatment. Successful use of LSD, MDMA, psilocybin, ketamine, and others, as therapeutic tools for these listed disorders, could be just the beginning of an entirely "new" type of medicine for other, as-yet-unconsidered illnesses.

• Anxiety Disorders
• Autism
• Obsessive-Compulsive Disorder
• Addiction
• Cluster Headaches

75. What are the anxiety disorders that are being experimentally treated with psychedelics?

As mentioned, there are ongoing studies with respect to MDMA-assisted treatment for PTSD. Other anxiety disorders being researched include social anxiety disorder, particularly with regard to patients who are autistic; end-of-life anxiety; anxiety associated with life-threatening illness. MDMA, LSD, psilocybin,

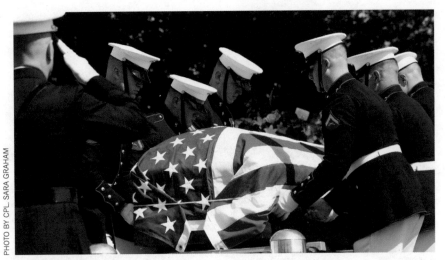

▲ **FIGURE 9.2**

According to *icasualties.org*, from 2001 into 2015 , there have been 2273 casualties of US military service personnel in the Afghanistan war, and since 2003, there have been 4494 casualties in Iraq. This is a total of 6767 US military fatalities over a span of 14 years.

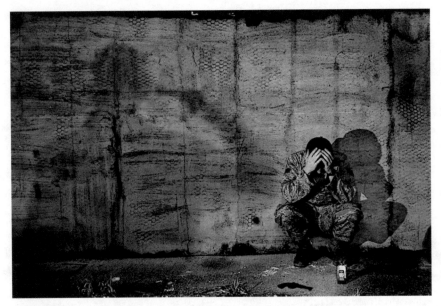

▲ **FIGURE 9.3**

According to John Isakson, Chairman of the US Senate Veteran Affairs Committee, an estimated 8,000 veterans of the US Armed Forces die by suicide each year. This is a total of approximately 112,000 suicides over the same span of 14 years (see caption for Figure 9.1), or 16 times the number of war casualties.

and cannabis are being researched for their potential to benefit therapy for some of these conditions.

76. Why are studies of PTSD so important?

Posttraumatic stress disorder is a far more serious condition than many of us realize. Most of us have reactions to memories of something hurtful that happened to us; we might have a nightmare occasionally, or we might develop an aversion to sitting with our back to the door, or we might detour our route in order to avoid a particular intersection where we'd had a near-fatal accident. These are all examples of mild posttraumatic stress. However, this type of stress manifests itself dozens—or even hundreds—of times over for patients with diagnosed PTSD. Often, a sufferer of chronic PTSD is unable to work, unable to maintain healthy relationships, unable to interact socially; many attempt or commit suicide.

Imaging studies such as fMRI show that "PTSD involves changes in the brain. Studies show that PTSD patients have decreased activity in the **hippocampus** and **prefrontal cortex** (brain areas associated with memory and learning) and increased activity in the **amygdala** (associated with fear)."—"Treating PTSD with MDMA-Assisted Psychotherapy," *http://www.mdmaptsd.org/images/ TreatingPTSD_brochure.pdf*

The amygdala activates the "fight or flight response" in the body; it triggers an alarm that throws the senses into overdrive to immediately determine whether a situation is "safe" or "unsafe." It does not reason, ponder, or plan—those are the jobs of the hippocampus and the prefrontal cortex. Normally, these parts of the brain communicate with each other naturally and easily.

For more details, please visit "Treating PTSD with MDMA-Assisted Psychotherapy" at

http://www.mdmaptsd.org/ images/TreatingPTSD_brochure.pdf

and "PTSD and the Brain" at

http://www.strengthofawarrior.org/ ptsd-and-the-brain/

However, traumatic stress disrupts the communication . . . The Thinking Brain cannot get the message through to the amygdala that the danger is over and it's okay to relax. The hippocampus cannot take the emotional information processed by the amygdala and store it away as a long-term memory. So your memories of trauma stay with you all the time, and you continue to feel as if you are in constant danger.

—"PTSD and the Brain," *http://www.strengthofawarrior.org/ ptsd-and-the-brain/*

PTSD is caused by such traumatic events as sexual assault, combat, torture, violent attack, childhood abuse, life-altering accidents, natural disasters, and other particularly stressful experiences. Here are a few quick facts about PTSD:

- Almost 7% of Americans suffer from PTSD at some point in their lifetime.
- Estimates vary, but approximately 1 in 7 to 1 in 5 veteran soldiers of the Iraq and Afghanistan wars are diagnosed with PTSD.
- Suicides among veterans account for 20% of all suicides in the United States.
- According to a 2006 report in *Psychological Bulletin* (published by the American Psychological Association), although men experience a greater number of traumatic events, women are more likely to experience the kind of violent traumatic event (sexual assault) that leads to PTSD.
- The *National Women's Study* (an extensive research project by the NIDA, published in 1997) reported that almost 31% of rape victims suffer from PTSD; 11% might have it for their entire lives.
- The US NIMH lists 1,318 clinical studies for PTSD and other anxiety disorders; of these, there are currently 16 studies that involve research with psychedelics MDMA, LSD, and psilocybin.
- One out of three PTSD sufferers do not respond to traditional treatment methods. Many of these people experience **delayed-onset** PTSD; the stress-causing trauma might have occurred a considerable length of time, possibly many years, before the onset of symptoms. These people have buried the trauma so deep in their psyche that traditional therapeutic approaches cannot tap into it.

77. How do the psychedelics compare with psychotherapeutic medicines that are currently being prescribed for PTSD?

Presently, the FDA approves two antidepressants for treatment of PTSD, the **selective serotonin reuptake inhibitor (SSRI)** medications sertraline and paroxetine; these medications relieve, somewhat, symptoms of depression and anxiety such as insomnia, inability to feel interest or joy, lack of concentration. These medicines are somewhat effective, but as mentioned about antidepressants in general, they merely mask symptoms, they do not cure. They will continue to be prescribed for a patient for as long as he or she needs relief from symptoms caused by PTSD—for many people this is years, for many others it is the rest of their lives. And, as can be heard on any television commercial advertising antidepressants, SSRIs come with a significant number of possible negative side effects: sexual dysfunction; high heart rate; interaction with anticoagulants (warfarin, aspirin, NSAIDs) caus-

DEFINITION

Selective serotonin reuptake inhibitors (SSRIs) are a class of compounds typically used as antidepressants in the treatment of major depressive disorders and anxiety disorders. SSRIs are believed to increase the extracellular level of the neurotransmitter serotonin by limiting its reabsorption into the presynaptic cell, increasing the level of serotonin in the synaptic cleft available to bind to the postsynaptic receptor.

https://en.wikipedia.org/wiki/Selective_serotonin_reuptake_inhibitor

ing increased risk of internal and intercranial bleeding; risk of suicidal behavior; discontinuation syndrome (painful physiological responses to discontinuation of the drug); and serotonin toxicity when taken in high doses or with multiple drugs.

Recall the description of the reuptake process in Chapter 3: normally, the serotonin is reabsorbed by the presynaptic neuron after the neurotransmitter has transmitted the neural impulse. SSRIs control the amount of serotonin in the synaptic cleft by inhibiting the reuptake process. Also from Chapter 3, recall that serotonin, a variant of tryptamine, controls moods such as depression, anxiety, pleasure, and contentment, and it significantly affects self-esteem.

78. How does MDMA help treat posttraumatic stress disorder?

Simply put, MDMA more or less reverses the activity in the brain that is caused by posttraumatic stress by significantly decreasing the brain activity in the left amygdala. Like SSRIs, it works to increase the level of serotonin in the synaptic cleft. However, instead of inhibiting a reuptake process, MDMA works by stimulating a massive release of stored serotonin from vesicles in the presynaptic membrane, which floods the synaptic gap and transmits the nerve impulse to the postsynaptic neurotransmitter.

MDMA's advantage over SSRIs is that it has the ability to *decrease the level of fear* built up in the amygdala *while increasing levels of trust, empathy, and positive feelings toward others.* This makes it possible for therapist and patient to achieve a stronger, more open connection and allows the patient to confront his or her personal trauma in a safe environment and in a nonthreatening way. Used in this manner, it is a *tool* to help the psychotherapist get to the root of the PTSD sufferer's trauma, thereby effecting a more thorough course of therapy to eventually overcome the disorder. A few facts about MDMA:

- Although MDMA is frequently called ecstasy, they are not the same. Substances sold on the street as ecstasy might contain MDMA, but they are "stepped on" with ketamine, caffeine, BZP, and other narcotics and stimulants—even toxic substances.
- In laboratory studies, pure MDMA has proven to be sufficiently safe for human consumption when taken in a clinical setting.
- Recreational MDMA (ecstasy) carries a greater risk of physical harm than classic psychedelics when taken in an uncontrolled manner. **Hyperthermia** can occur through prolonged physical exertion in a hot environment together with **dehydration**; such circumstances are classic in dance clubs. The effects of hyperthermia include liver and kidney failure and cerebral edema. Ecstasy can also cause **hyponatremia**, which is a condition that also involves the kidney and leads to increased water retention and associated decreased serum sodium, which in turn leads to nausea, weakness, fatigue, confusion, seizures, and coma.

- Deaths and incidents of physical harm are attributed to ecstasy, but there have been no reported deaths from pure MDMA administered clinically.

79. What are end-of-life anxiety disorder and anxiety from life-threatening illness?

Perhaps because it is inherent in human nature to fear death, as one approaches the end of one's life, anxiety is a common struggle. Although it's perfectly natural to fear something we've never faced before, for many, the anxiety becomes overwhelming and symptoms such as shortness of breath, nightmares, and pain develop, and characteristics of clinical depression become unmanageable:

- Lack of enjoyment of people or activities one used to enjoy
- Major changes in sleeping or eating habits
- Ideation of suicide
- Panic attacks (see definition)
- Estrangement or withdrawal from one's family, friends, and environment
- Disassociation or out-of-touch feeling with one's self, as though being "on the outside, looking in"

According to the Academy of Psychosomatic Medicine,

Psychiatric problems and issues commonly seen at the end of life include anxiety symptoms and anxiety disorders, depressive symptoms and depressive disorders, delirium and other cognitive disorders, suicidal ideation, consequences of low-perceived family and other social support, personality disorders or personality traits that cause problems in the setting of extreme stress, questions of capacity to make informed decisions, grief and bereavement, and general and health-related quality of life. Spiritual and religious issues, including both personal faith and relationship to a community of believers, are important for most people. Good end-of-life care requires explicit attention to these matters.

—*http://www.apm.org/papers/eol-care.shtml*

Clinical depression affects approximately 20% of people diagnosed with a terminal disease such as cancer or AIDS. Frequently, clinical depression is not diagnosed and goes untreated or patients receive only palliative care.

80. How can psychedelics assist with end-of-life anxiety and life-threatening illnesses such as end-stage cancer?

There is a rich history of using psychedelics to assist patients with the existential issues associated with dying, and much of the work in this field was done by Stanislav Grof and Joan Halifax in the 1960s. The spiritual awakening achieved by ingesting LSD or psilocybin or peyote seems to be particularly appropriate at the end of life. A study published in 2011 by Charles Grob, Professor of Child and Adolescent Psychiatry at the Harbor-UCLA Medical Center in Torrance, California, was the first published clinical study since the early 1970s. It explored the possibilities of using psilocybin to ease the fear of death and enrich patients' final stage of life with spiritual comfort. The Harbor-UCLA study became the first psychedelic treatment with terminally ill patients since the early 1970s. All of the patients in the study had end-stage cancer and were experiencing unremitting anxiety. Using a double-blind, placebo-controlled method, the study demonstrated that psilocybin-assisted psychotherapy reduced psychospiritual anxiety, depression, and physical pain for these patients.

Panic attacks are intense periods of pounding heart or accelerated heart rate, sweating, trembling or shaking, sensations of shortness of breath or smothering, feeling of choking, chest pain or discomfort, nausea or abdominal distress, feeling dizzy, unsteady, light-headed or faint, fear of losing control or going crazy.— Center to Advance Palliative Care; *https://www.capc.org/fast-facts/145-panic-disorder-end-life/*

Studies show that psychiatric morbidity [the incidence of both physical and psychological deterioration as a result of a psychological condition] in the setting of terminal illness is exceptionally high. The prevalence of delirium in terminal cancer and AIDS patients ranges from 30%–85%, and the prevalence of clinically significant depression ranges from 20%–50%.

—Academy of Psychosomatic Medicine; *http://www.apm.org/papers/eol-care.shtml*

Another clinical study of psilocybin for sufferers of cancer is currently under way at Johns Hopkins University by Roland Griffiths and his team. In this study, 44 patients are being treated with psilocybin-assisted psychotherapy. It is similar to the Harbor-UCLA study, but the Johns Hopkins efforts will be to work with early-stage as well as late-stage cancer patients. It is hoped that findings will show that psilocybin can relieve the pain associated with cancer in addition to improving quality of life and helping patients overcome the anxiety and existential crises associated with their diagnosis of cancer.

At NYU, a similar pilot study is in progress that will assess the efficacy of psilocybin on psychosocial distress, particularly with regard to anxiety associated with advanced cancer. This study involves 32 participants and the dosage of psilocybin is intended to be a higher measure than that used in the Harbor-UCLA study.

81. What is social anxiety disorder?

Just as PTSD is an extreme form of mild traumatic stress, social anxiety disorder (SAD) is a severe manifestation of the typical anxiety many people experience when they are in social situations, meeting new people, or in large crowds. A few facts about SAD:

- Sufferers of SAD live in deep fear of social situations.
- SAD causes considerable difficulty in maintaining an ability to function in many aspects of daily life.
- Physical symptoms often accompany SAD: excessive blushing, sweating, trembling, heart palpitations, awkward speech patterns such as stammering or rapid speech, and nausea.
- Anxiety is usually triggered by situations of either a real or a perceived threat of being judged.

 At the Heffter Institute website you can find descriptions of the three psilocybin and cancer studies undertaken at NYU, Harbor-UCLA, and Johns Hopkins and links to the published articles;

http://www.heffter.org/index.htm

 There are interesting videos (each approximately 10 minutes long) of interviews with volunteers from the three studies mentioned;

http://www.heffter.org/video.htm

"Psilocybin at the End of Life," with Charles Grob, MD, discusses his research in this area and can be seen at

https://www.youtube.com/watch?list=SP4F 0vNNTozFTJCv1cvvUyB11CRR62uee8&v=t WeEp0S1AAQ

The Johns Hopkins Psilocybin Research Project is discussed by Roland Griffiths at

https://www.youtube.com/watch?v= lbRbMavHm-8

A video lecture about LSD-assisted treatment studies, "LSD-Assisted Psychotherapy in the Treatment of Anxiety Secondary to Life Threatening Illness," with Peter Gasser, MD, can be viewed at

https://www.youtube.com/watch?list=SP4 F0vNNTozFTJCv1cvvUyB11CRR62uee8& v=3k8mOG0aDXM

- SAD is the most common anxiety disorder and one of the most common psychiatric disorders.
- 12% of American adults have experienced SAD.

82. How are SAD and autism linked for research with psychedelics?

Perhaps the most significant characteristic of autism is the diminished ability to interact socially. Children who are near the severe end of the autistic spectrum might not respond when spoken to and often avoid eye contact with other people. Although certain necessary social skills might be cultivated as they grow to adulthood, autistic children do not have the ability to interpret tones of voice, gestures, and facial expressions, so they cannot empathize with what others are thinking or feeling. The attitude of being in "their own little world" can invite ridicule and even bullying from other children, thus aggravating the tendency for these children to develop SAD as they mature.

Autistic adults often suffer from anxiety, trauma, depression, and social adaptability challenges and are at greater risk for psychological disorders, especially SAD, which intensifies the already substantial number of social challenges that autistic adults encounter. A few facts about autism:

- ASD varies significantly in character and severity.
- ASD occurs in all ethnic and socioeconomic groups and affects every age group.
- In 2014, it was estimated that 1 out of 68 children in the United States will have some degree of ASD.
- Males are four times more likely to have an ASD than females.

So, people who are autistic are challenged by SAD as a characteristic of their primary disorder; research using psychedelics as a tool to treat SAD is hoped to be beneficial for autistic patients as well.

"The multilevel effects of MDMA on brain circuits, monoaminergic neurotransmitters, and neurohormones that have been studied extensively in autistic individuals suggest that further study of the effects of MDMA in autistic populations is warranted."—"MDMA-Assisted Therapy: A New Treatment Model for Social Anxiety in Autistic Adults"; *http://dx.doi.org/10.1016/j.pnpbp.2015.03.011*

83. What is Obsessive-Compulsive Disorder?

Obsessive Compulsive Disorder (OCD) is a disorder of the brain and behavior. OCD causes severe anxiety in those affected. OCD involves both **obsessions** and **compulsions** that take a lot of time and get in the way of important activities the person values.—*https://iocdf.org/about-ocd/*

Much like SAD, obsessive-compulsive disorder (OCD) varies in intensity from individual to individual, and it is frequently misunderstood as simply a strange idiosyncrasy that makes people wash their hands frequently or line things up in a specific order. In truth, OCD is a very disabling and difficult-to-treat condition. Described as a "Bully in the Brain," OCD grabs onto a thought or image and will not let it go. The brain "gets stuck," paralyzing the sufferer's ability to move forward and on to other thoughts or endeavors.

You might remember, from childhood, skipping along a sidewalk and avoiding the cracks, chanting, "Step on a crack and you'll break your mother's (or teacher's, brother's, etc.) back." Avoiding cracks in the linoleum or the sidewalk and, yes, repeated handwashing, reciting certain numerical combinations, ordering and reordering items are well-known symptoms of OCD; however, with OCD, the crux of these habits is that they are rooted in fear and anxiety. The Bully in the Brain insists that certain rituals be performed over and over again before it will allow the fear to dissipate. The Bully in the Brain is just like the bully on the playground: it will want more and more from an individual as time goes by; reordering the socks on the clothesline twice becomes reordering three, four, and five times or else the threat of great danger (breaking your mother's back) looms constantly. A few facts about OCD:

- OCD affects approximately 2.3% of the world population; 2.2 million Americans.
- It is rare for symptoms to occur in people over the age of 35.
- 50% of people who develop OCD do so before the age of 20, roughly 30% develop symptoms as children.
- OCD affects males and females about equally.
- OCD symptoms can fluctuate in severity at different times and can even appear intermittently.

84. What is it about obsessions that makes them part of a disorder?

Obsession: A persistent and disturbing intrusion of, or anxious and inescapable preoccupation with, an idea or feeling especially if known to be unreasonable
—*http://unabridged.merriam-webster.com/unabridged/obsession*

DEFINITION

Obsessions are thoughts that occur repeatedly and uncontrollably. In current vernacular, an obsession is not necessarily a bad thing. The term "obsessed" has come to be used rather loosely; one is "obsessed" with her smartphone, his video games, a new song, a personality followed on Twitter, a philosophy or "cause," or any number of things or ideas. However, these are more casual—and not quite accurate—interpretations of the word *obsessed*.

In the context of OCD, an obsession is much more serious and detrimental. Per the formal definition given, the thought or impulse that lodges in the mind is a "disturbing intrusion" on an individual's ability to function in an ordinary fashion from day to day; the "inescapable preoccupation" stems from fear and anxiety. OCD obsessions tend to be grave concerns, and the fears and anxieties center on losing control, germs and contamination, life-threatening diseases, perfectionism, sexual thoughts, religion, superstitions, and potential harm to self or others.

85. What are compulsions?

Compulsion: an irresistible impulse to perform an irrational act; a driving by force, power, pressure, or necessity —*http://unabridged.merriam-webster.com/unabridged/compulsions*

DEFINITION

Compulsions are repetitive behaviors enacted by an irresistible impulse. People with OCD follow their compulsions to alleviate their obsessions; they rely on their compulsions to temporarily escape the thoughts that obsess them. Compulsive behaviors are a way of trying to control fear; if a certain compulsion is repeated a certain number of times or in a certain order, the OCD sufferer feels "safe." Compulsions are time consuming in that they are repeated over and over until the individual feels anxiety and fear lessen; they get in the way of important activities such as work, school, and even pleasant social occasions.

86. Are psychedelics being researched to assist in the treatment of OCD?

Anecdotal reports suggest that many sufferers with obsessive-compulsive disorder frequently show a spontaneous remission of symptoms, sometimes lasting several weeks, when they take LSD or magic mushrooms; however, clinical research did not resume after the '70s until 2006, when a double-blind, placebo-controlled pilot study was conducted at the University of Arizona, led by Dr. Francisco Moreno. Participants in the study were nine patients who had severe OCD that had not responded to traditional treatments. Psilocybin was shown to substantially reduce OCD symptoms in several of the patients, one for several weeks after the treatment.

"This study shows a potential breakthrough treatment for obsessive-compulsive disorder, a recalcitrant disease that is the fourth most common outpatient psychiatric problem."—The Heffter Research Institute; *http://www.heffter.org/research-pocd.htm*

NOTE

Dr. Moreno's study was published in the *Journal of Clinical Psychiatry* in 2006; it is available online through *PubMed.gov*: "Safety, Tolerability, and Efficacy of Psilocybin in 9 Patients with Obsessive-Compulsive Disorder."

PRACTICAL TIP

http://www.ncbi.nlm.nih.gov/pubmed/17196053?dopt=AbstractPlus

Research of this approach to OCD is still young, but there is certainly more to come in this field in the future.

The Heffter-Zürich Research Center has begun preclinical studies focused on researching the effects of psilocybin on the neuroreceptors in the human brain. It is believed that there might be significant data to encourage the use of psilocybin for the treatment of obsessive-compulsive spectrum disorders (OCSDs), which include anorexia and other eating disorders, as well as OCD.

Data being collected with these scans and studies will show the normal levels of 5-HT2A receptors in the brain and how psilocybin affects them. These data will create a baseline for clinical studies that will follow up on the pilot study at the University of Arizona, mentioned previously.

87. Can psychedelics be used to treat depression?

Research into the possibilities of psychedelics being used in many ways and for many disorders is in its infancy. However, psychedelics have been shown to reduce depression, perhaps indirectly: they promote feelings of closeness between patient and therapist, which enhances therapy for depression; they increase relaxation and reduce paranoia; and drugs such as MDMA also have the important characteristic of being able to reduce the fear of recalling of traumatic memories, which in itself alleviates depression.

The effects of MDMA on raising mood and improving feelings of well-being are very clear and well documented. Theoretically, MDMA could be a potent serotonin enhancer to treat depression, but there is very little empirical clinical information regarding the effects of MDMA on depressed patients, and until clinical studies have successfully investigated therapeutic applications for MDMA, this question cannot yet be answered with confidence. The rise in mood, or "high," during recreational use of MDMA by depressed people is often followed by a subsequent depressed mood and other associated unpleasant psychological and physiological "hangover" effects, which, at present, are deterrents to such theory.

Although clinical studies for psychedelic-assisted therapy for depression and mood disorders are too young to have yielded definitive results, brain imaging studies (PET, fMRI, MRS, ERP) have demonstrated that psilocybin has the ability to elevate mood.

88. What are cluster headaches?

Cluster headache is a neurological disorder characterized by recurrent, severe headaches on one side of the head, typically around the eye . . . belonging to a group of primary headache disorders, classified as the **trigeminal autonomic cephalalgias**.

—*https://en.wikipedia.org/wiki/Cluster_headache*

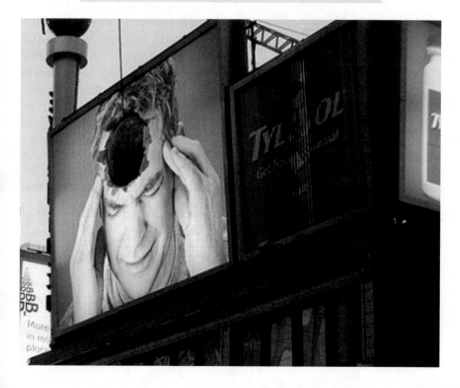

Cluster headaches are a little-known malady that affect only one or two people out of every 1000. They are more intensely painful than migraines; in fact, they are considered to be *the #1 most painful medical condition known to medical science.* The term "cluster" refers to the grouping and episodic nature of the repeated headache attacks, which occur several times a day over long periods of time—several months is not unusual—followed by periods of remission.

The excruciating pain radiates into the jaw and teeth on the same side of the head as the headache pain and is accompanied by nasal congestion and runny nose, contracting pupils and tears, and facial drooping or flushing. A few facts about cluster headaches:

- They are also known as "suicide headaches" because the pain is so intense that sufferers often threaten to commit suicide rather than bear the pain—and some have.
- Women who experience cluster headaches claim that the pain is worse than the pain of giving birth.
- Cluster headaches affect about 1 million Americans.
- Cluster headache sufferers are mostly males (90%).
- Cluster headaches cannot be relieved by painkillers.

89. Which psychedelic compounds are being researched to treat cluster headaches?

In 1998, there was a posting on an Internet bulletin board by a man who reported that his use of LSD had prevented his usual cluster headache cycles. He had successfully experimented on himself and posted that he planned to continue using LSD as a treatment. As happens with such bulletin boards, more reports of self-experimentation with psychedelics began to appear. Postings, discussions, and experiments continued into 2001, and soon an Internet-based support group called Clusterbusters was founded by Bob Wold.

NOTE

The authors interviewed 53 cluster headache patients who had used psilocybin or lysergic acid diethylamide (LSD) to treat their condition. Twenty-two of 26 psilocybin users reported that psilocybin aborted attacks; 25 of 48 psilocybin users and 7 of 8 LSD users reported cluster period termination; 18 of 19 psilocybin users and 4 of 5 LSD users reported remission period extension. Research on the effects of psilocybin and LSD on cluster headache may be warranted.
—"Response of Cluster Headache to Psilocybin and LSD," by A. Sewell, J. Halpern, and H. Pope. 2006. *Neurology*, 66(12):1920–1922.

By 2004, large numbers of anecdotal reports were popping up on the Clusterbusters website about the usefulness of recreational classical psychedelics for relieving cluster headache pain. It seemed that small, "subpsychedelic" doses of LSD or magic mushrooms helped the painful headaches disappear for many weeks or even months afterwards. Armed with a significant number of anecdotal data, Bob Wold approached MAPS and asked them to evaluate these reports. A subsequent review of these cases by Andrew Sewell, John Halpern, and Harrison Pope has led to a new study, which is still under development.

In addition, Halpern, together with Torsten Passie at Medizinische Hoschule Hannover in Germany, had also been developing a nonhallucinogenic version of LSD: 2-Bromo-LSD, or "BOL." BOL has been used in place of LSD in subsequent studies.

90. How can psychedelics be helpful in the treatment of addictions?

Recall from previous chapters that early studies of LSD by Humphry Osmond and Abram Hoffer focused on alcohol dependence. Although results from these studies are hardly conclusive— particularly as there has since been some criticism of mid-20th century protocols—there has been continued interest in studying psychedelics for their use in addiction therapies. Interestingly, the impetus for much of the current work in this

 PRACTICAL TIP
More information about Clusterbusters can be found at their website; *https://clusterbusters.org/*

 PRACTICAL TIP
The results of the Halpern–Passie study are available at *http://ck-wissen.de/ckwiki/ images/1/14/IHS_IHC_2009_ BOL_Halpern.pdf*

 ON THE WEB
There are two Clusterbuster videos featuring Bob Wold, who discusses cluster headaches and various studies with psychedelics to treat them. The first includes footage of a sufferer enduring a cluster headache episode. The second is a more recently published video (2013) that includes more detail—including description of other current, quite invasive procedures being used to treat cluster headache sufferers.

https://vimeo.com/15967891

https://www.youtube.com/watch?v= Jv1lG417LKg2013

A video lecture on "The Use of LSD, Psilocybin, and Bromo-LSD for the Treatment of Cluster Headaches," featuring Torsten Passie, MD, can be viewed at *https://www.youtube.com/ watch?v=FNonSMghN40*

"Psilocybin-Assisted Treatment for Alcohol Dependence"
is a 30-minute video featuring Dr. Michael Bogenschutz,
who discusses studies of LSD, psilocybin, and other psychedelics for addiction
therapy; *https://www.youtube.com/
watch?v=pAdmGMceP-4*

ON THE WEB

The US NIH *ClinicalTrials.gov*
website lists "A Double-Blind Trial
of Psilocybin-Assisted Treatment
of Alcohol Dependence" study
by Michael Bogenschutz, MD, of New York
University. This study is currently about to
enter Phase II, once participants have been
recruited. *https://clinicaltrials.gov/ct2/
show/NCT02061293*

NOTE

"MAPS-sponsored researchers
are collecting observational data
for the first prospective ibogaine
outcome studies in order to contribute to the growing scientific literature
about ibogaine as a treatment for drug addiction." —*http://www.maps.org/research/
ibogaine-therapy#accordion31*

NOTE

field is the Osmond and Hoffer hypothesis that the psychedelic experience is life-style altering. There is much evidence from different sources to support the theory that addictions such as alcoholism can be mitigated by behavioral changes on the part of the addict, and use of classic psychedelics can facilitate such changes.

The mystical, or spiritual, experience prompted by psychedelics could be key in such behavioral changes. As noted in Chapter 6, Bill Wilson, founder of AA, supported the use of LSD by alcoholics because it was his belief that LSD could help people awaken to a spiritual connection with their Higher Power.

Ibogaine is a naturally occurring psychoactive from the rainforest iboga shrub in western Central Africa. It has proven to be effective in the treatment of opiate addictions such as heroin, and it has been noted that ibogaine reduces withdrawal symptoms and cravings for opiate substances. There are independent ibogaine treatment centers in Mexico and New Zealand for patients undergoing this therapy.

Psilocybin-assisted therapy for tobacco addiction has been under study by a team led by Matthew W. Johnson, PhD, at John Hopkins University. As with studies on alcohol dependence, the crux of the "cure" lies in the modification of behavior by a spiritual awakening through the use of the psychedelic. Published in 2014, this study is the first scientific study of the use of a psychedelic as a therapeutic tool to conquer smoking. The study was **open-label**, which means that the volunteers were aware that they were receiving the psilocybin; therefore, definitive conclusions cannot be drawn; however, the success rate indicates that subsequent research is called for. Johnson and colleagues intend to begin a follow-up study that will involve randomized, control-conditioned experiments and brain-scan imaging.

This chapter has explored some of the current research into the use of psychedelics as tools to assist with psychotherapy. You might have noted that we have not discussed or mentioned cannabis. There is so much information and media attention about medical marijuana that it deserves its own chapter, so we have devoted Chapter 10 to "Cannabis."

"How a Schizophrenic Drug Addict Reclaimed His Life with Iboga" by Luke Sumpter is the real-life story of a man who had been diagnosed with schizophrenia that did not respond to antipsychotics and antidepressants. In his long quest for some relief from his illness, he eventually tried ibogaine and claims that it is a successful treatment.

http://reset.me/story/how-a-schizophrenic-drug-addict-reclaimed-his-life-with-iboga/

"Study results . . . indicate that 12 out of 15 volunteers receiving psilocybin-assisted psychotherapy for smoking cessation were able to remain smoke-free after a six-month follow-up"—"Psilocybin Mushrooms Help People Quit Smoking and Other Addictions," Michael W. Johnson et al., *Journal of Psychopharmacology*, 2014.

For details of Johnson's study, visit *http://reset.me/story/psychedelics-treating-tobacco-addictions/*

Cannabis

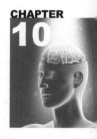

Although listed as a Schedule 1 substance, cannabis is far less harmful than other compounds; however, because of its classification, it has taken decades for independent researchers to acquire it for study. As you will read in this chapter, the potential uses for cannabis, or medical marijuana, are many; governmental obstruction to legalize its use is considered by most experts to be "absurd."

91. What about medical marijuana?

The term **medical marijuana** refers to using the whole unprocessed marijuana plant or its basic extracts to treat a disease or symptom. *https://www.drugabuse.gov/publications/drugfacts/marijuana-medicine*

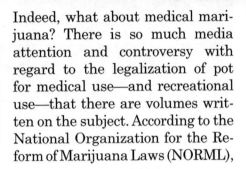

DEFINITION

Indeed, what about medical marijuana? There is so much media attention and controversy with regard to the legalization of pot for medical use—and recreational use—that there are volumes written on the subject. According to the National Organization for the Reform of Marijuana Laws (NORML),

Cannabis is . . . one of the most investigated therapeutically active substances in history. To date, there are approximately 22,000 published studies or reviews in the scientific literature referencing the cannabis plant and its cannabinoids, nearly half of which were published within the [past] ten years according to . . . PubMed Central, the US government repository for peer-reviewed scientific research.

—http://norml.org/component/zoo/category/recent-research-on-medical-marijuana

There are many hundreds of active components in cannabis, but two in particular stand out as important: **delta-9 tetra-hydrocanibinol (THC)**, which is generally considered to be the principal chemical that produces the psychoactive, psychedelic effect of the high; and **cannabidiol (CBD)**, which is the chemical that produces the more relaxed, dreamy effect.

A federally sponsored research report from NIDA is available online at *https://www.drugabuse.gov/publications/research-reports/marijuana*.

PRACTICAL TIP

Although the FDA has not recognized or approved the whole botanical marijuana plant as medicine, scientific study of the chemicals in marijuana, called **cannabinoids**, has led to two FDA-approved medications. These are synthesized cannabinoid chemicals in pill form. *—https://www.drugabuse.gov/publications/drugfacts/marijuana-medicine*

NOTE

Our knowledge of the medicinal uses for cannabis continues to grow, although research into cannabis has been difficult because of restrictions on its use, hindered by the NIDA and the DEA since the 1970s when it was listed as a Schedule 1 drug.

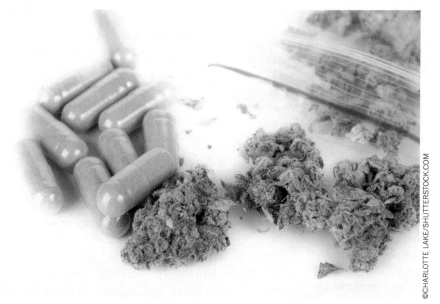

▲ **FIGURE 10.1**
Cannabis to pills.

©CHARLOTTE LAKE/SHUTTERSTOCK.COM

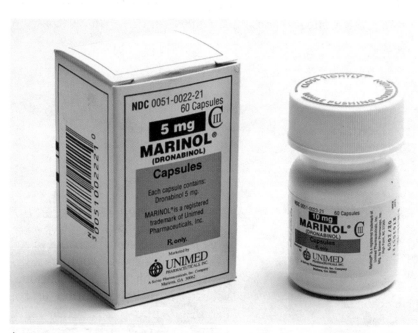

COURTESY OF THE DEA MUSEUM

▲ **FIGURE 10.2**
Marinol®, (synthetic THC, or dronabinol) has been marketed since 1999 (placed on
Schedule III) for the control of nausea and vomiting caused by chemotherapy used in the
treatment of cancer and to stimulate appetite in AIDS patients.

NIDA has a supply of marijuana for its own research, and NIDA scientists have been conducting preclinical and clinical trials with regard to

- autoimmune diseases (diseases that weaken the immune system):
  - HIV/AIDS
  - multiple sclerosis (MS), which causes gradual loss of muscle control
  - Alzheimer's disease, which causes loss of brain function, affecting memory, thinking, and behavior
- inflammation
- pain
- seizures
- substance use disorders
- mental disorders

92. What is "Uncle Sam's Pot Farm"?

The 1970 Controlled Substances Act (CSA; see Chapter 7) gave the DEA the responsibility of regulating the cultivation

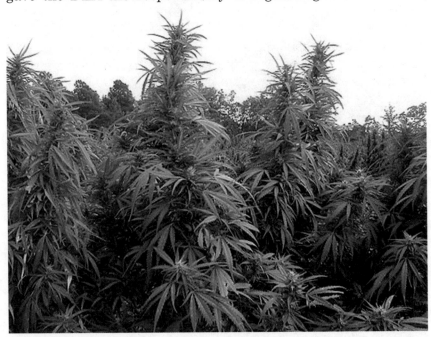

▲ FIGURE 10.3
Close up of just a few marijuana plants at Uncle Sam's Pot Farm; actual crop sizes vary from 1.5 to 6.5 to 12 acres, depending on demand.

of marijuana for research purposes through issuing licenses. To date, the DEA has issued only one license to grow marijuana for research: to the University of Mississippi, for use exclusively by NIDA.

 A brief televised interview with Dr. Mahmoud ElSohly, who oversees the marijuana farm at the University of Mississippi, can be seen at *https://www.youtube.com/watch?v=IEJf2-TdU68*

The federal government's pot farm rests on 12 acres at "Ole Miss" and includes an indoor lab facility with controls for light, temperature, humidity, and CO_2 concentration. The outdoor fields are secured by double fences, guards, and video monitoring and handle the "cultivation, growing, harvesting, analyzing, and storing of research-grade cannabis," according to the NIDA webpage.

Uncle Sam's pot farm grows a variety of strains of the marijuana plant, with different amounts of the two primary chemicals. One strain might be 70% THC and 30% CBD, another might be 50/50 percent of each, and so on.

93. What is NIDA's role in the research on marijuana?

As a government agency, NIDA's efforts are, of course, on behalf of the government's stance on controlled substances. Note that the name of the agency is the National Institute on Drug Abuse (subtitled The Science of Drug Abuse & Addiction), rather than a less prejudicial name such as "National Institute on Drug Sciences" or the like. As might be expected, the majority of these studies have some bias toward what is *bad* about marijuana.

NIDA sponsors research by awarding grants for studies *on the federal level*. Most of these studies investigate the use of individual cannabinoid chemicals derived from the marijuana plant; in other words, the studies do not use the whole plant because the FDA, as mentioned, has not approved the plant as medicine. It is a typically tangled web of government bureaucracies: the DEA dispenses licenses, but (thus far) only to NIDA; NIDA grows pot, but only for its own research; NIDA offers grants (and marijuana and its chemical derivatives), but only to federally approved proposed studies.

There are mandatory criteria to be satisfied in order to qualify as a federally approved pot grower, and these are several difficult "hoops" to jump through, including DEA registration,

"As part of its mandate to study drug abuse and addiction and other health effects of both legal and illegal drugs, NIDA funds a wide range of research on marijuana; its main psychoactive ingredient, delta-9-tetrahydrocannabinol (THC); and chemicals related to THC . . ."

"NIDA has provided and continues to provide funding for research related to therapeutic uses of cannabinoids, as it pertains to its mission."

https://www.drugabuse.gov/drugs-abuse/marijuana/marijuana-research-nida

For more detail on government requirements for growing weed for research, explore "Production, Analysis, and Distribution of Cannabis and Related Materials" at

https://www.fbo.gov/index?s=opportunity&mode=form&id=a9add8776134243fdae0a06ee07d1b4c&tab=core&_cview=1.

Dr. Wilson Compton briefly discusses NIDA's concerns with regard to legalization of marijuana and how shifts in policy affect societal concerns of a community and the impact of marijuana on health and behavior, particularly on the adolescent brain.

https://www.drugabuse.gov/drugs-abuse/marijuana/marijuana-research-nida.

facility specifications, a DEA- and FDA-approved storage vault, and other stipulations.

NIDA's concerns with regard to researching medical marijuana extend beyond scientific exploration of THC and CBD; as a division of the National Institutes for Health, NIDA has a responsibility to the public to ensure the safety and efficacy of cannabis as medicine and must consider all of the ramifications of legalizing marijuana: Is it addictive? Is it a "gateway" drug? How does use of marijuana affect one's ability to work, drive, perform at school, interact socially?

94. Is NIDA-sponsored research the only research being conducted?

Independent, privately funded medical marijuana research has been stonewalled for decades because the DEA has not allowed researchers to grow their own pot and because the legal acquisition of marijuana for research is tied up in so much red tape. The MAPS organization, however, has battled the DEA for over a decade to gain access to or to grow whole-plant marijuana in their efforts "to demonstrate the safety and efficacy of botanical marijuana as a prescription medicine for specific medical uses to the satisfaction of the US Food and Drug Administration" (*http://www.maps.org/research/mmj#accordion51).*

On June 22, 2015, the US Department of Health and Human Services (HHS) announced "the elimination of the Public Health Service (PHS) review of non-federally funded research protocols involving marijuana and the utilization of the existing Food and Drug Administration (FDA) Investigational New Drug (IND) process for drug development."

This policy shift could portend an increase in the amount of research to be conducted because it removes a stumbling block of redundancy in the approval process for private research.

 Medical marijuana advocates and researchers are celebrating a surprise decision by the Obama administration to scrap reviews that delayed—sometimes for years—private and state-funded research into marijuana's medical value . . . Researchers will no longer need to submit proposed pot studies to the US Public Health Service for review, ending a hurdle that does not exist for research of other drugs listed as Schedule I substances . . .—*U.S. News & World Report*, June 22, 2015.

Since 1999, researchers seeking to study marijuana needed to obtain permission from PHS to purchase marijuana from the National Institute on Drug Abuse (NIDA), which maintains a monopoly on the supply of marijuana for research in the United States. Now, researchers with Food and Drug Administration (FDA) clearance can request marijuana directly from NIDA without the additional PHS review process.

—*http://www.maps.org/index.php?option=com_content&view= category&id=110&Itemid=636*

95. What are some medical conditions that cannabis could benefit?

In addition to the list of preclinical and clinical trial topics being researched by NIDA scientists (see Q. 89), NORML writes,

Modern research suggests that cannabis is a valuable aid in the treatment of a wide range of clinical applications. These include pain relief—particularly of neuropathic pain (pain from nerve damage)—nausea, spasticity, glaucoma, and movement disorders. Marijuana is also a powerful appetite stimulant, specifically for patients suffering from HIV, the AIDS wasting syndrome, or dementia. Emerging research suggests that marijuana's medicinal properties may protect the body against some types of malignant tumors and are neuroprotective

—*http://norml.org/marijuana*

96. Can cannabis be used as a tool to assist psychotherapy?

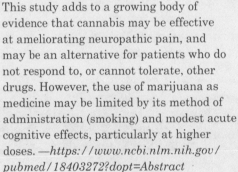

To understand the nature of the delays and the frustrations encountered by MAPS (and other researchers), view a timeline of the events of a MAPS study that was first conceived in 2009 and that, after six years, is still awaiting DEA approval. *http://www.maps.org/ index.php?option=com_content&view=category &id=248&Itemid=593*

A report titled "A Randomized, Placebo-Controlled, Crossover Trial of Cannabis Cigarettes in Neuropathic Pain" states,
This study adds to a growing body of evidence that cannabis may be effective at ameliorating neuropathic pain, and may be an alternative for patients who do not respond to, or cannot tolerate, other drugs. However, the use of marijuana as medicine may be limited by its method of administration (smoking) and modest acute cognitive effects, particularly at higher doses. —*https://www.ncbi.nlm.nih.gov/ pubmed/18403272?dopt=Abstract*

Research on marijuana's potential use in psychiatry is very limited, however, what study there is revolves around the chemistry of the THC and the CBD. As mentioned, the CBD provides the dreamy, relaxing effect of the cannabis plant. It is theorized that CBD might have an antipsychotic effect and could act as an antidepressant or anxiolytic (antianxiety) drug. This is an area that deserves a great deal more research.

The aforementioned study being developed by MAPS focuses on marijuana to assist in the treatment of symptoms of PTSD in US veterans. The study will be a placebo-controlled, triple-blind, randomized crossover pilot study. Five different strains of marijuana (five different percentage ratios of CBD to THC), will be tested in 76 US veterans who have chronic, treatment-resistant PTSD. This study will explore whether smoking or inhaling vaporized marijuana can help reduce PTSD symptoms that have not responded positively to other medications or to psychotherapy.

Additional research is being conducted at the Center for Medicinal Cannabis Research, at the University of California through a legislated state program. Although the bulk of these studies are clinical trials focusing on the medical uses for cannabis, there is a study by Igor Grant, MD, with regard to psychiatric and neurocognitive effects of cannabis on behavior.

Medical marijuana is the recent "hot topic" in psychedelic science. Many states have passed laws to legalize dispensaries and a few have legalized the recreational use of the botanical, whole-plant marijuana. It seems likely that more states will follow suit and open the doors for further research and that the drug might eventually be dropped from Schedule I status. This is an exciting but sadly out-of-date concept—that a centuries-old herb, proven by ancient shamans of various religions and tribes to be effective medicinally in a variety of ways, will be the "newest" analgesic and might also quell nausea, spasticity, glaucoma, and movement disorders.

Part IV of our exploration of psychedelic drug therapy presents thoughts and discussion on the future of psychedelics in assisting psychotherapy.

PRACTICAL TIP

For a complete list of possibly treatable maladies and details of medical marijuana's potential benefits, read a report titled "Emerging Clinical Applications for Cannabis & Cannabinoids: A Review of the Recent Scientific Literature, 2000—2015" at *http://norml.org/pdf_files/NORML_ Clinical_Applications_for_Cannabis_and_ Cannabinoids.pdf*

ON THE WEB

A slide-show presentation of Dr. Grant's study, "Neuropsychiatric Effects of Cannabis," can be viewed at *http://www.cmcr .ucsd.edu/images/pdfs/AAAS2015.pdf*

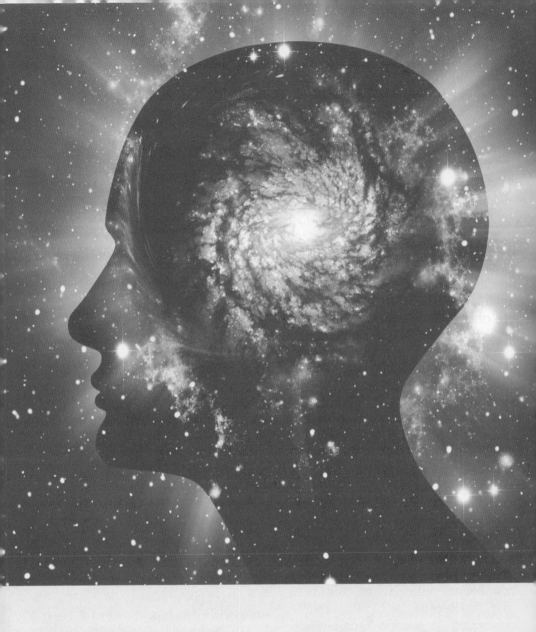

PART FOUR

The Future of Psychedelics

In these chapters we discuss whether psychedelics can, indeed, become useful as tools for psychotherapy. Chapter 11 evaluates the potential for these drugs to become legally prescribed medicines someday. Safety issues are discussed in Chapter 12, and Chapter 13 encourages a better understanding of the viable use of psychedelic drugs to assist psychotherapy. These chapters are followed by a Summary.

The Future for Psychedelic-Assisted Psychotherapy

CHAPTER 11

97. Do psychedelics really have a future in modern psychotherapeutic medicine?

Although promising research was halted and in limbo for several decades, today we are beginning to see progress in contemporary psychedelic research. The number of studies being proposed and developed is increasing, numerous clinical and neurophysiological studies are being published every week, and studies that are currently being conducted continue to show positive results.

Functional neuroimaging is the use of neuroimaging technology to measure aspects of brain functions to understand the relationship between activity in certain brain areas and specific mental functions. It is primarily used as a research tool in cognitive neuroscience, cognitive psychology, neuropsychology, and social neuroscience.

Modern imaging techniques applied to the study of the brain have expanded understanding of the physiological processes behind the subjective psychological effects of psychedelic drugs. Functional Magnetic Resonance Imaging (fMRI) images of the brain on psilocybin, for example, graphically traced and measured the subjective psychological effects of psilocybin when a subject was recalling pleasing memories. This is a breakthrough for psychotherapy because it proves that psychedelics can open the brain to repressed emotional memories. Being able to represent graphically what heretofore had been merely theorized is a huge step forward.

ON THE WEB

fMRI images of the brain on placebo and on psilocybin are shown as figures and as Power-Point presentations in a study titled "Neural Correlates of the Psychedelic State as Determined by fMRI Studies with Psilocybin," by Dr. Robin Carhart-Harris et al., available at *http://www.pnas.org/content/109/6/2138.full* Brain-imaging research that includes fMRI and MEG imaging with psilocybin and fMRI with MDMA has been conducted by Dr. Robin Carhart-Harris and Professor David Nutt. A video presenting their research can be watched at *http://www.psychedelicscience.org/18-conference-workshops/48-brain-imaging-studies-with-psilocybin-and-mdma.html*

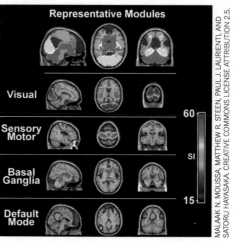

Representative Modules

Visual

Sensory Motor

Basal Ganglia

Default Mode

60

SI

15

> **FIGURE 11.1**
These images of the "resting" (not focused on a specific task) brain show four functional neural networks: the visual (yellow), sensory/motor (orange), basal ganglia (red) cortices, and default mode network (maroon). The "resting state" approach is used to determine whether the brain's functional organization is altered in neurological or psychiatric diseases. Courtesy of wiki commons.

The authors do not have a crystal ball and cannot foretell the future, but psychedelics are the perfect drugs to assist psychotherapy: They are short acting and, so, can be administered for a single session of therapy. They have no significant dependency issues. They are completely nontoxic at doses proposed for clinical use and are considerably safer than antipsychotics and antidepressants. They are shown to reduce depression. They enhance motivation for therapy by increasing feelings of closeness between patient and therapist, increase relaxation, and reduce paranoia. They stimulate new ways of thinking to explore entrenched problems.

When the pharmacological effects of psychedelic drugs are combined with effective and expertly guided psychotherapy, a new way of treating old psychiatric problems is at hand. Under the influence of drugs such as MDMA, LSD, ayahuasca, and psilocybin—used with care and supervision—patients can confront their memories of abuse, and, with their therapist, explore and repackage the sensory aspects of a traumatic event and *put that memory away* in the compartmentalized area of their past, where it belongs.

98. Which of the psychedelic compounds seem to have the best potential for continued research?

In addition to the characteristics of other psychedelics, MDMA is also able to reduce the fear of remembering traumatic events from one's past. This allows the patient to focus objectively on the memory itself without being overwhelmed by negative feelings. So, it seems that MDMA might be the most beneficial drug to assist psychotherapy and, therefore, will perhaps emerge as the most popular psychedelic for research.

Also, as seen in Chapter 9, MDMA is already being studied in connection with anxiety disorders such as PTSD and SAD and ASD, so it would seem that success in these areas will make MDMA a front runner as choice of drug for future work.

Psilocybin's effects and characteristics make it also a drug conducive to research, particularly for end-of-life anxiety, and it has also been used extensively for brain imaging studies.

99. Which seem closest to achieving legal status?

We have recently seen the legalization of medical marijuana in the form of two FDA-approved capsules or pills. The next goal is to work for the legalization of botanical, whole-plant marijuana so that researchers do not have to wait for years for study protocols to be approved and for delivery of marijuana from NIDA. As we learned in Chapter 10, medical marijuana, thus far, is being used to treat medical conditions. It's use in psychotherapy has yet to be studied.

MDMA is the focus of current study for several disorders, so it more than likely would be legalized sooner than LSD, psilocybin, or ayahuasca, if, indeed, it is legalized at all.

100. Is it possible that psychedelics can not only treat, but possibly cure?

Psychedelics are not "medicines"; one dose of LSD or psilocybin or MDMA is not going to solve a deeply rooted psychological issue or rid one of anxiety forever. These drugs are meant to be used as *tools* to assist the psychotherapist and patient to work together effectively, with trust and empathy. An open-minded, fear-dismissed psyche engaging with an experienced therapist to uncover the reality of past trauma, confront it, and evaluate it from an expanded and existential perspective can help a patient overcome feelings of powerlessness. Patients can eventually feel more in control of their actions and feelings and can move forward with their lives, leaving the past behind. For many, this would be a "cure."

Safety Issues, Side Effects, and Ethics

CHAPTER 12

101. Is there a downside to psychedelic-assisted therapy?

There is no such thing as an entirely "safe" drug. As seen in Chapter 7, even caffeine can be toxic. In this volume, the authors are not attempting to condone recreational drug use or to suggest that MDMA or any other illegal substance is completely safe. Although classic psychedelics produce very few physiological changes, there are valid concerns

Remember that MDMA is not a classic psychedelic; it's an entirely synthesized chemical, and does not derive from natural plants, mold, or fungi.

NOTE

that MDMA, for instance, can induce a low mood as its effects wear off, that it can induce preexisting anxiety and depression in susceptible individuals, that it produces unwanted acute side-effects such as bruxism (teeth gnashing and grinding), hyperthermia, and dehydration; very rare cases of uncontrolled recreational use can cause an idiosyncratic adverse reaction that may even be fatal.

However, in clinical use, the side effects are reduced because pure MDMA is used, and dosage, room temperature and other environmental conditions, and the patient's vital signs are monitored.

102. Are there ethical considerations with regard to psychedelic-assisted therapy?

In so far as "ethics" and "laws" frequently go hand in hand, one should consider that because the drugs are illegal, it is not ethical to promote their use. However, the medical community of doctors, researchers, and therapists has well-established structures of external regulatory control, powerful and empowered patient groups, clear lines of accountability, ethics committees, and other rules for clinical governance and health and safety; these are provided to ensure the appropriate and ethical concerns of such therapy.

But for all drugs, whether used recreationally or prescribed, the public deserve to be given a realistic risk-to-benefit ratio and accurate reporting of relative risks as they participate in clinical trials. If, at some point, successful trials earn approval from the FDA, psychedelics will become legal for use in psychotherapy, and risks will be stipulated. However, as we've learned with regard to clinical trials procedures, those days are still a long way off.

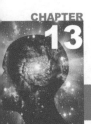

CHAPTER 13

Opening the Door to a Better Understanding

103. How do enlightened consciousness and spirituality play a part in psychotherapy?

This book has included many mentions of the entheogenic properties of the psychedelics; heightened consciousness, spirituality, becoming "at one" with the universe, expanding the mind, and so forth. So, what does that have to do with psychiatry?

There is no easy answer to that question. Does it mean that therapy should be conducted with an open Bible on a side table and sessions should begin and end with a prayer? Certainly not. That is to confuse religion with spirituality. Spirituality as meant here is an awareness of being part of something wider, larger, in a quite cellular way.

We have also discussed the empathogenic characteristics of psychedelics—the ability for therapist and client to connect on an empathetic level. This is easier to understand because empathy is a typical human emotion, an ordinary state of consciousness. The entheogenic awareness—the "God within and without" consciousness—is nonordinary, felt perhaps by only a few spirited saints and monks who live among us.

Quantum physics tells us that everything is made up of particles that have energy and move in a wavelike motion. An enlightened interpretation of this state theorizes that if all things are in

"The Implications of Consciousness Research for Psychiatry, Psychology, and Psychotherapy" by Stan Grof is a comprehensive discussion of the phenomenon of "consciousness," which, after all, is not generated by the brain but by an energy within and without; https://www.youtube.com/watch?list=SP4F0vNNTozFTJCv1cvvUyB1 1CRR62uee8&v=iPg5jeNwXLs

ON THE WEB

a form of perpetual energetic movement, then the energy is in us and in everything around us. In an ordinary consciousness state we might not perceive this, but in a nonordinary state—for example, having ingested a perception-altering drug—this energy can be experienced. This energy transcends the self's ego and opens a new dimension: spirituality, an awareness and trust that all experiences and things work together. The fabric of the present is the past and the future; understanding this, a patient is more likely to overcome traumatic events of the past and to recognize his or her own "divinity."

104. How can this research achieve greater acceptance?

As we read in Chapter 7, the notoriety achieved by psychedelic drugs in the 1960s and '70s was incredibly distorted and sullied by their proliferation into the mainstream. The recreational abuse of what were potentially neuroscientific breakthroughs was played up by the media, and medical and psychiatric research efforts were barely mentioned in the media at all.

"The reverberation caused by the social *opinion* of what something is *imprints* us even if we know better."—Lakshmi Narayan

In order to alter misconceptions about these substances, it will be necessary to erase the image of the frying egg from the public mind. Brain imaging studies can graphically illustrate what is really going on in the brain on drugs.

"This is your brain on drugs" was a 1987 televised commercial of an egg (the brain) frying in a frying pan (on drugs) as part of a nationwide antidrug campaign sponsored by Partnership for a Drug-Free America: *https://www.youtube.com/watch?v=ub_a2t0ZfTs*

According to the study from which Figure 13.1 was captured, "This supports our idea that psilocybin disrupts the normal organization of the brain with the emergence of strong, topologically long-range functional connections that are not present in a normal state." The key word in that sentence is "functional"; the brain remains functional, the connections made are insightful beyond the connections ordinarily made. The brain does not get "fried," nor does it turn to mush or become dysfunctional. This is the kind of credible, significant discovery that the media should be bringing to public attention.

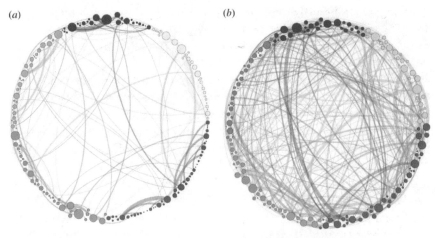

(a) (b)

▲ FIGURE 13.1
This is your brain on psilocybin. Two drawings that represent an fMRI study on 15 healthy individuals' brains. (a) The stable brain activity in a healthy brain that received a placebo. (b) On psilocybin, many different brain regions become strongly connected, indicating expansion and processing of nonordinary conscious thought.
SOURCE: "Homological Scaffolds of Brain Functional Networks," G. Petri, P. Expert, F. Turkheimer, R. Carhart-Harris, D. Nutt, P. J. Hellyer, F. Vaccarino, *Interface* 11: 101(2014).
http://rsif.royalsocietypublishing.org/content/11/101/20140873.full.pdf+html
© 2014 The Authors. Published by the Royal Society under the terms of the Creative Commons Attribution License http://creativecommons.org/licenses/by/4.0/, which permits unrestricted use, provided the original author and source are credited.

"Repositioning Psychedelics in the Public Mind," Brad Burge, Arianne Cohen, and Lakshmi Narayan:

ON THE WEB

https://www.youtube.com/watch?list=SP4 F0vNNTozFTJCv1cvvUyB11CRR62uee8& v=vFOhGh1AANk

A true story cannot be retracted, and what happened when psychedelics merged with the hippie culture cannot be undone; however, a new story can be told. A story of credible scientists and researchers and practitioners and their brain imaging and clinical studies must now capture the attention of the media in order to undo the damage caused by "the earlier story." Decades from now these drugs—plants and mold and fungi and synthetic MDMA—will be the norm. We will look back on their negative history as being no more consequential than "Clark Stanley's Snake Oil Treatment" and other patent medicines. It is time to restructure the Schedules set forth by the CSA, and it is time to remove redundant and absurd obstructions to independent, nonfederally funded research.

Summary

"So I consider LSD to be of some value to some people,
and practically no damage to anyone."

—Bill Wilson

We have learned that the heydays of hippies and legal drugs were detrimental to a developing aspect of medical and psychiatric research that is both viable and valuable. It is irrefutable that psychedelic substances have a great deal to tell the neuroscientific

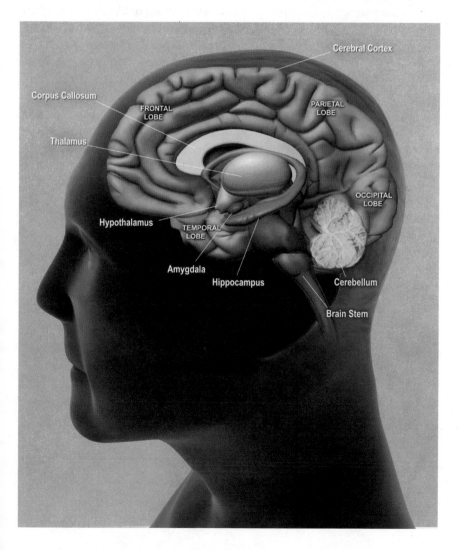

community about the brain, behavior, and altered states of consciousness, and it is unfortunate that years have passed that could have been devoted to this research.

After discussing the history of research into psychedelics, it should be apparent that the time has come to renew and revisit the vast possibilities that these drugs can offer to those populations of our society who suffer anxieties and stress and mental health disorders to debilitating degrees. These substances are not and were never meant to be recreational drugs; they are medical agents, pharmacological compounds designed for the medical and psychiatric professions. That was the original intent for their use, and it is the intent of present-day researchers to establish a place for these drugs as sound medical and psychiatric tools.

We gave a rudimentary lesson on the neurotransmitter pathways in the brain and introduced some of the terms used in neuroscience. We also mentioned that with ever-advancing technologies such as brain-imaging scans, scientists have the ability to represent graphically the physiological changes in the brain manifested by psychedelic compounds. Seeing which parts of the brain are influenced by these drugs increases understanding of their effects. It's no longer necessary to rely on anecdotal accounts and try random doses of this or that psychoactive; the research community has become more knowledgeable and sophisticated in its approach to clinical trials, and further efforts will be based on data gained and considered irrefutable.

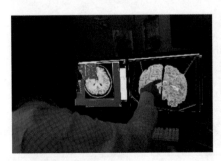 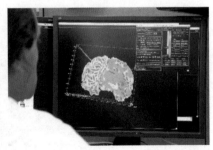

▲ **FIGURE S.1 AND S.2**
Analyses of brain imaging data.
SOURCE: Images courtesy of the National Institute of Mental Health.

We have learned that the psychedelic drugs—as any drugs—handled inappropriately, can be dangerous. It is important to emphasize that when used in a clinical setting by reputable therapists and doctors, these drugs have very few physiological effects, which are quite mild; most antidepressants and antipsychotics legally on the market today have side effects that are far more uncomfortable or even life threatening. The authors strongly believe that the psychedelics should remain in the hands of professional, licensed doctors and therapists; set and setting are of utmost importance when using these substances, and tested protocols—dosage, length of time between doses, and so forth—should be followed; and full consideration should be given to whether more standard approaches to therapy have failed and patients are truly "blocked."

States of bliss, enlightenment, and spiritual emergence are valid mental states experienced by many people. That they are difficult to comprehend and describe with our current medical language does not mean they do not exist, any more than suggesting the mental state of love doesn't exist. The spiritual, uplifting, consciousness-expanding properties of these substances cannot be denied. However, it was these characteristics that appealed so powerfully to recreational users in the '60s. How naïvely headstrong to believe that the world's turning might alter direction toward love and peace if everyone could just "take a pinch of psychedelic." It was not to be—not then and not now. But perhaps, at some point in the future—when PTSD victims can be relieved of their suffering, when autistic adults are able to interact sociably without discomfort, when end-stage cancer victims find that they can let go of pain and addicts can let go of their addictions—perhaps, in the course of treating these afflictions, a universal, enlightened-consciousness mindset will begin to prevail, and as Huxley put it, "Love as the primary and fundamental cosmic fact" will finally be the rule that keeps the world turning.

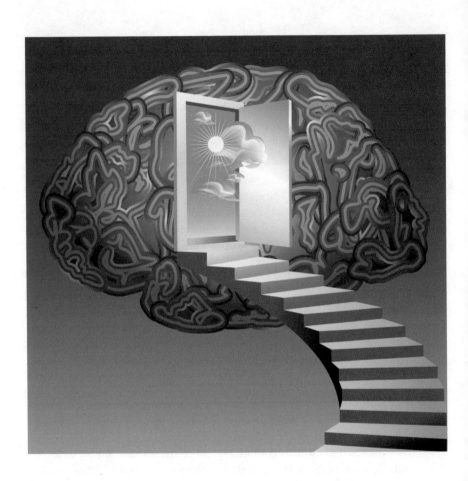

Appendix

URLs to Videos and Suggested Readings

CHAPTER 1 Videos

"Psychedelic Drugs–The Unexplained, Part I" at *http://www .youtube.com/watch?v=XtB8SUlaM8g*

"What is a drug?" at *https://www.udacity.com/course/ viewer#!/c-ps001/l-233544439/e-233198861/m-233198862*

"Psychoactive and psychotropic" at *https://www.udacity.com/ course/viewer#!/c-ps001/l-233544439/m-233198872.*

"Exploring aspects of drugs" at *https://www.udacity.com/ course/viewer#!/c-ps001/l-233544439/m-233198866.*

CHAPTER 1 Suggested Readings

Classes of psychotropic drugs and psychiatric disorders at *http://www.nimh.nih.gov/health/publications/mental-health- medications/index.shtml*

CHAPTER 2 Videos

Lucy in the Sky with Diamonds by John Lennon & Paul McCartney (1967) at *http://www.youtube.com/watch?v =ZqXmBy1_qOQ*

Rare footage from 1950s of live subject's reaction to taking LSD at *https://www.youtube.com/watch?v=BTjRi0x2Cyg&list =PL709ufoAtf4fvTCm2m6bSRptH2JUHMAHE&index=9*

National Geographic Explorer documentary on LSD at *https:// www.youtube.com/watch?v=14WtwJTwuWg*

Erowid ("Earth Wisdom") website at *www.erowid.org/chemicals/*

Alexander (the godfather of MDMA) and Anne Shulgin at *http://www.youtube.com/watch?v=9kDl-V5RuQo*

CHAPTER 2 Suggested Readings

The "Bibles" of psychoactive substances by Alexander and Anne Shulgin:

PiHKAL (Phenethylamines i Have Known and Loved)

TiHKAL (Tryptamines i Have Known and Loved)

CHAPTER 3 Videos

"The Human Brain" at *http://www.youtube.com/watch?v =1imN6oc_YtU*

"How Does the Brain Work?" (Nova 1080pHD) at *http://www .youtube.com/watch?v=lhIJbIX1_D0*

"The Universe Inside Your Head" at *http://www.brainfacts.org/ brain-basics/neural-network-function/articles/2013/the -universe-inside-your-head/*

Slideshow of the way the nervous systems interact at *http:// www.mayoclinic.org/brain/SLS-20077047?sl=?&slide=6*

3-D animation of neurotransmitters crossing the synaptic cleft at *www.youtube.com/watch?v=90cj4NX87Yk*

Two narrated lessons with greater detail about the synaptic action: *http://www.youtube.com/watch?v=p5zFgT4aofA http://www.youtube.com/watch?v=TevNJYyATAM*

Detailed explanation of agonists and antagonists at *http://www .youtube.com/watch?v=uXREQnFGHGA*

God Is in the Neurons explores the chemistry of the brain, its neurotransmitters, and neural connections to self-awareness, emotions, consciousness, and spirituality at *http://www .youtube.com/watch?v=oPEdDcs_8ZQ&feature=youtu.be*

CHAPTER 3 Suggested Readings

"Entheogens and Entactogens" by Nicholas Novak in *NeuroSoup* at *http://www.neurosoup.com/entheogens-and-entactogens/*

CHAPTER 4 Videos

"How Do Psychedelic Drugs Work in the Brain?" with Dr. Robin Carhart-Harris at *http://www.youtube.com/watch?v =jT5dZDnJ6J4*

"Psychedelic Drugs–The Unexplained, Part II" at *http://www .youtube.com/watch?v=rH5MQYdae5Y*

CHAPTER 5 Suggested Readings

History of ancient mushroom use in the Erowid Vaults at *http://www.erowid.org/plants/mushrooms/mushrooms_ history.shtml*

Timeline of medical cannabis use from 2900 B.C. to the present at *http://medicalmarijuana.procon.org/view.timeline.php? timelineID=000026*

By the creator of LSD, *LSD: My Problem Child: Reflections on Sacred Drugs, Mysticism and Science* by Albert Hofmann

CHAPTER 6 Videos

LSD Experiment filmed in 1955—"Schizophrenic Model Psychosis Induced by LSD-25" at *http://www.youtube.com/ watch?v=M7fOuPTZtWI*

"Psilocybin-Assisted Treatment for Alcohol Dependence" at *http://www.maps.org/conference/ps13michaelbogenschutz/*

Famous 1955 experiment in which Humphry Osmond administered mescaline to British parliament member Christopher Mayhew, not shown at the time it was filmed, at *https://www .youtube.com/watch?v=Eh8IBLs61_M*

Huxley's theories and his mescaline experience. *http://www .youtube.com/watch?v=mbI4f1WvN9w*

A two-part video, *"Stan Grof About His LSD Experience and Research,"* is quite interesting:
Part 1: *http://www.youtube.com/watch?v=5ig3eU_oDS0*
Part 2: *http://www.youtube.com/watch?v=-tSRHStwOPU*

An interview with Reverend Randall Laakko, participant in the Good Friday Experiment at *http://www.youtube.com/watch?v=DxDZW6n69-0*

A movie trailer titled *Walter Pahnke and the Good Friday Experiment* at *http://www.youtube.com/watch?v=G6mlyt34-gc*

Timothy Leary's Trip Thru Time is an image-rich slideshow at *http://timothyleary.org/#1*

CHAPTER 6 Suggested Readings

Pass It On, Bill Wilson's official AA biography

Acid Dreams: The Complete Social History of LSD: The CIA, the Sixties, and Beyond by Martin A. Lee and Bruce Shalin; selected pages available at *http://www.levity.com/aciddreams/samples/capthubbard.html*.

Online biography of Al Hubbard, a.k.a. "Captain Trips" and the "Johnny Appleseed of LSD," at *http://www.rense.com/general28/dshwo.htm*

Pahnke's first-hand account of the Marsh Chapel experiment at *http://www.erowid.org/entheogens/journals/entheogens_journal3.shtml*

CHAPTER 7 Videos

CIA Mind Control Operation MK ULTRA, full-length ABC News documentary filmed in the 1970s, at *http://www.youtube.com/watch?v=2t-L26MjwRo*

"The Five Most Shocking CIA Experiments of Project MK Ultra" at *http://www.youtube.com/watch?v=7ff24-xGrSI*

Brief video also titled "CIA Mind Control Operation MK ULTRA," at *http://www.youtube.com/watch?v=i46RI2twVao*

CHAPTER 7 Suggested Readings

"Serotonin, and the Past and Future of LSD" by David E. Nichols, PhD, at *www.maps.org/news-letters/v23n1/v23n1_p20-23.pdf*

Article about the Beat Generation at *http://www.online-literature .com/periods/beat.php*

Fascinating stories of psychedelic history can be found in *Acid Dreams. The Complete Social History of LSD: The CIA, the Sixties, and Beyond* by Martin A. Lee and Bruce Shalin, New York: Grove Press, 1992. (See also Chapter 6, url to selected pages.)

CSA schedule levels and lists of all the controlled substances at *http://www.deadiversion.usdoj.gov/schedules/#list* or, at *http://www.fda.gov/regulatoryinformation/legislation/ ucm148726.htm* (this FDA site provides the complete text of the Controlled Substances Act, and the schedules are more complete).

CHAPTER 8 Suggested Readings

Recent psychedelic research publications, *PubMed.gov* or *ClinicalTrials.gov*

Past preclinical and clinical studies in database archive *World Wide Web Psychedelic Bibliography* at *http://www.maps.org/ resources/psychedelic-bibliography*

CHAPTER 9 Videos

"MDMA-Assisted Psychotherapy for PTSD: Current Research with Veterans, Firefighters, and Police Officers," by researchers Michael Mithoefer, MD, and Annie Mithoefer, BSN at *https:// www.youtube.com/watch?v=-QozbvrjwMY*

Interviews with volunteers from three psilocybin and cancer studies undertaken at NYU, Harbor-UCLA, and Johns Hopkins at *http://www.heffter.org/video.htm*

"Psilocybin at the End of Life," with Charles Grob, MD at *https://www.youtube.com/watch?list=SP4F0vNNTozFTJCv1c vvUyB11CRR62uee8&v=tWeEp0S1AAQ*

Johns Hopkins Psilocybin Research Project is discussed by Roland Griffiths at *https://www.youtube.com/watch?v =lbRbMavHm-8*

"LSD-Assisted Psychotherapy in the Treatment of Anxiety Secondary to Life Threatening Illness," with Peter Gasser, MD at *https://www.youtube.com/watch?list=SP4F0vNNTozFTJCv 1cvvUyB11CRR62uee8&v=3k8mOG0aDXM*

Experiences of ASD patients after they took MDMA, in their own words, at *http://www.psychedelicscience.org/18-conference-workshops/49-findingsfrom-a-collective-case-study-on-the-mdmaecstasy-experiences-of-adults-on-the-autismspectrum.html*

Image of a PET scan of a brain on psilocybin at *http://www .heffter.org/research-hz.htm*

"Neurobiology of Psychedelics–Implication for Mood Disorders"; neuroimaging studies (PET, fMRI, MRS, ERP) of the effect of psilocybin on emotion regulation and discusses its potential as an antidepressant. *http://www.psychedelicscience.org/18-conference-workshops/67-neurobiologyof-psychedelics-implication-for-mood-disorders.html*

Cluster headache lecture; footage of a sufferer enduring a cluster headache episode at *https://vimeo.com/15967891*

More recent (2013) cluster headache lecture with more detail—including description of other current quite invasive procedures being used to treat cluster headache sufferers at *https://www .youtube.com/watch?v=Jv1lG417LKg2013*

"The Use of LSD, Psilocybin, and Bromo-LSD for the Treatment of Cluster Headaches" featuring Torsten Passie, MD, at *https:// www.youtube.com/watch?v=FNznSMghN40*

"Psilocybin-Assisted Treatment for Alcohol Dependence" featuring Dr. Michael Bogenschutz and discussion of LSD, psilocybin, and other psychedelics for addiction therapy at *https://www.youtube .com/watch?v=pAdmGMceP-4*

"How a Schizophrenic Drug Addict Reclaimed His Life with Iboga," a case study by Luke Sumpter at *http://reset.me/story/ how-a-schizophrenicdrug-addict-reclaimed-his-life-with-iboga/*

CHAPTER 9 Suggested Readings

"Treating PTSD with MDMA-Assisted Psychotherapy" at *http://www.mdmaptsd.org/images/TreatingPTSD_brochure.pdf*

"PTSD and the Brain" at *http://www.strengthofawarrior.org/ptsd-and-the-brain/*

An illustrated poster titled "Treating PTSD with MDMA-Assisted Psychotherapy" at *http://www.mdmaptsd.org/infographic.html*

Three psilocybin and cancer studies undertaken at NYU, Harbor-UCLA, and Johns Hopkins and links to the published articles at *http://www.heffter.org/index.htm*

"MDMA-Assisted Therapy: A New Treatment Model for Social Anxiety in Autistic Adults" at *http://dx.doi.org/10.1016/j.pnpbp.2015.03.011*

"Safety, Tolerability, and Efficacy of Psilocybin in 9 Patients with Obsessive-Compulsive Disorder." *http://www.ncbi.nlm.nih.gov/pubmed/17196053?dopt=AbstractPlus*

"Response of Cluster Headache to Psilocybin and LSD," by A. Sewell, J. Halpern, and H. Pope. 2006. *Neurology*, 66(12): 1920–1922.

"Psilocybin Mushrooms Help People Quit Smoking and Other Addictions," Michael W. Johnson et al. at *http://reset.me/story/psychedelics-treating-tobacco-addictions/*

CHAPTER 10 Videos

Dr. Mahmoud ElSohly, who oversees "Uncle Sam's Pot Farm" at the University of Mississippi at *https://www.youtube.com/watch?v=IEJf2-TdU68*

NIDA's concerns about legalization of marijuana with Dr. Wilson Compton at *https://www.drugabuse.gov/drugs-abuse/marijuana/marijuana-research-nida*

"Neuropsychiatric Effects of Cannabis" slideshow at *http://www.cmcr.ucsd.edu/images/pdfs/AAAS2015.pdf*

CHAPTER 10 Suggested Readings

Cannabis; federally sponsored research report from NIDA at *https://www.drugabuse.gov/publications/research-reports/marijuana*

"Production, Analysis, and Distribution of Cannabis and Related Materials" at *https://www.fbo.gov/index?s=opportunity&mode=form&id=a9add8776134243fdae0a06ee07d1b4c&tab=core&_cview=1*

Timeline of events of a MAPS study awaiting DEA approval at *http://www.maps.org/index.php?option=com_content&view=category&id=248&Itemid=593*

"A Randomized, Placebo-Controlled, Crossover Trial of Cannabis Cigarettes in Neuropathic Pain" at *https://www.ncbi.nlm.nih.gov/pubmed/18403272?dopt=Abstract*

"Emerging Clinical Applications for Cannabis & Cannabinoids: A Review of the Recent Scientific Literature, 2000—2015" at *http://norml.org/pdf_files/NORML_Clinical_Applications_for_Cannabis_and_Cannabinoids.pdf*

CHAPTER 11 Videos

"Neural Correlates of the Psychedelic State as Determined by fMRI Studies with Psilocybin" PowerPoint presentations by Dr. Robin Carhart-Harris et al. at *http://www.pnas.org/content/109/6/2138.full*

Brain-imaging research that includes fMRI and MEG imaging with psilocybin and fMRI with MDMA at *http://www.psychedelicscience.org/18-conference-workshops/48-brain-imagingstudies-with-psilocybin-and-mdma.html*

CHAPTER 13 Videos

"The Implications of Consciousness Research for Psychiatry, Psychology, and Psychotherapy" with Stan Grof at *https://www.youtube.com/watch?list=SP4F0vNNTozFTJCv1cvvUyB11CRR62uee8&v=iPg5jeNwXLs*

"This is Your Brain on Drugs," a 1987 televised commercial at *https://www.youtube.com/watch?v=ub_a2t0ZfTs*

"Repositioning Psychedelics in the Public Mind," with Brad Burge, Arianne Cohen, and Lakshmi Narayan at *https://www.youtube.com/watch?list=SP4F0vNNTozFTJCv1cvvUyB11CRR62uee8&v=vFOhGh1AANk*

Index

depression, treatment for, 100–101
designer drugs, 12
dimethyltryptamine (DMT), 18, 19
dissociatives, 13, 15
dopamine, 26, 27
double-blind, placebo-controlled,
  randomized study, 56, 75–76
Drug Enforcement Administration
  (DEA), 67
dysthymic disorder, mood stabilizers
  for, 8

E

ecstasy. *See* 3,4-methylenedioxy-
  methamphetamine (MDMA)
Ellis, Henry Havelock, 42
empathogens. *See* entactogens
end-of-life anxiety disorder, 93,
  94–95
endogenous substances, 27
entactogens, 30
entheogen, 28–29
  psychedelic drugs as, 29–30
epinephrine, 26
ergot (*Claviceps purpurea*), 39–40
euphoriants, 17
European Commission, 83
exogenous substances, 27

F

Federal Analogue Act, 12
first-generation antipsychotics, 9
Food and Drug Administration
  (FDA), 61, 67, 111
  approval of drugs, 74
  clinical study, 74
Functional Magnetic Resonance
  Imaging (fMRI), 116
functional neuroimaging, 116

G

generalized anxiety disorder (GAD),
  antianxiety medications for,
  8–9
Ginsberg, Allen, 47
Grof, Stanislav, 47, 53–54

H

hallucinations, 13, 15
hallucinogens, 13
  vs. psychedelics, 14–16

Harbor-UCLA study, 94
Harvard Psilocybin Project, 55
Heffter, Arthur Carl Wilhelm, 42
Heffter Research Institute, 83
heroin, 67
Hoffer, Abram, 48
Hoffman, Abbie, 47
Hofmann, Albert, 42–45
  LSD, discovery of, 43–45
Hubbard, Alfred, 47
  as "Captain Trips", 51–52
Huxley, Aldous, 47, 49–51
hyperthermia, 92
hyponatremia, 92

I

ibogaine, 19–20, 104
illusions, 14, 15
in vitro, 74
inebriants, 17
International Federation for Internal
  Freedom (IFIF), 58
Investigational New Drug (IND), 111
involuntary nervous system. *See*
  autonomic nervous system

J

Jimson weed, 38

L

L-DOPA, 27–28
Leary, Timothy, 47, 58–60
  experiment with LSD, 58–59
  involvement in psychedelics, 55
  research contribution, 54–55
legal ecstasy. *See* 2C-B
Lewin, Louis, 42
lysergic acid diethylamide (LSD),
  19, 67
  Alfred Hubbard called as "Captain
    Trips", 51–52
  available in psychotherapy, 45
  discovery of, 42–45
  Huxley first try, 50–51
  Timothy Leary first experiment
    with, 58–59

M

magic mushrooms. *See* psilocybin
major depressive disorder, mood
  stabilizers for, 8

lysergic acid diethylamide
(LSD), 19
psilocybin, 19
tryptamines, 17

U

Uncle Sam's pot farm, 108–109
US Controlled Substances Act, 12
US Department of Health and
Human Services (HHS), 111
US Drug Enforcement
Administration (DEA),
12, 61, 67
US government, role in psychedelic
research, 63–64

V

vesicles, 25
voluntary nervous system. *See*
somatic nervous system

W

War on Drugs, 68
Web Tryp. *See* US Drug Enforcement
Administration